4 WEEKS TO A
NEW YOU
& NEW LIFE

YOUNGER; STRONGER, SLIMMER LIFESTYLE.

BY EVA SUNDENE

THE SCANDINAVIAN HEALTH & BEAUTY MANUAL

Independently Published
Printed in the United States of America, First Edition 2020

Eva Sundene, evasundene.com

About the Author

Eva Sundene is a Norwegian writer, a well-known innovator, lecturer and educator for all aspects of lifestyle, health, beauty, spa, slimming and body shaping.

She established the first lifestyle magazine in Scandinavia, Shape- Up, at the start of the eighties. She was chief editor, and the magazine was the trendsetter in the fields of aerobics, nutrition and fitness until the late nineties. After this, she needed more challenges, and then became the leading expert on spa concepts and spa education in Norway.

In 2011, she decided to move to the Canary Islands in Spain to get more out of life and have more time to enjoy her passion: Writing!

She is really living out all her favourite activities on the beautiful island of Fuerteventura. Her company Slankonline.com has online courses about lifestyle, slimming, health, anti-ageing, and beauty.

She says, "I love my active lifestyle here, and I can assure you that I have tested all that I recommend to you. I believe that all women can be beautiful in their own way, if they just make an effort and have the know-how. Turn the clock back and look and feel marvelous. I know this book can give you the tools you need to transform, so please give yourself a chance to feel younger, slimmer, more vibrant and beautiful by following my advice. I know they work firsthand."

Disclaimer

The Author and Publisher have tried to be as accurate as possible   in creating this book. The content is based on my personal experiences, meanings, and know-how. I assume no responsibility for errors, omissions, or contrary interpretation of the subject. This is a practical lifestyle guide, but there are no guarantees of individual results. Readers should rely on their own judgment about their individual circumstances and to act accordingly. This book is an inspiration and how-to guide that provides general health information. The book's content is not a substitute for professional medical care, diagnosis, or treatments. If you are in doubt of what is right for you, always ask you physician for advice.

evasundene.com

Table of Content

Table of Content

Table of Content

Table of Content

Table of Content

To my beloved daughter Vibeke, my son Christopher, my precious grandchildren, and great-grandchildren! Ida Emilie, Joachim, Preben and Mathias: You are all part of my heart, my past, present and the future. I love all of you forever and ever.

Love from Mimi Eva

Chapter 1

FOREVER YOUNG - THE LIFESTYLE

How are you really feeling about getting older? Are you accepting it, but not exactly rejoicing in the process? Honestly, you are probably like most of us and feel slightly afraid of what is going to happen as you pass each new birthday. Will you slowly deteriorate and get wobbly in both body and mind? Will you gradually change into a different person and become a little old lady with lots of aches and pains? In the Western world, we have been victims of such a negative view of the ageing process for years!

Ageism - worse than sexism?

Honestly, we are brainwashed by the extreme admiration of youth in media, advertising, fashion and the world of beauty in general. We look at taller-than-normal anorexic teenagers with heavy, freaky makeup on huge Bambi-eyes who are trying to look grown-up and sophisticated as they walk the runway or try to look seductively out of glossy magazine pages. But I am extremely glad that it's starting to change.

Age is shameless

Telling someone your age is no longer like swearing in church. Lots of the cosmetic companies and magazines are using forty and fifty-year-old plus models, as this age group is more important to consumers than younger models. It is a fact that the richest Western consumers are older, and of course they need to be pampered, not just accepted. Money talks...

So, whatever your age is, be proud of it. You have survived with flying colours so far, and you still have a long way to go, places to see, people to meet. You have to be fit for the fabulous future you have waiting for you. You have to feel happy with your looks and be willing to invest time and effort in yourself. This book is your guide to the very best version of you!

Don't worry, be happy...

I love that melody because for me that's what life is about. Taking one day at a time. Living in the now. Doing the best, you can in every way without being a perfectionist with sky-high stress levels. Don't worry, be happy that you are still around, and hopefully in reasonably good health. Be extremely grateful for each new and healthy day you have on this planet. Be so grateful that you do a great job keeping in shape and having the best health you can by making a conscious effort for yourself. The best choice is to not only accept that ageing is part of living, but to learn how to combat the negative effects of life's natural wear and tear.

Restore and reverse

Are you scared of the visibly increasing signs of aging you see in the mirror? Welcome to the club of women afraid to get old. Or is it welcome to the club of women who have accepted it and given up the fight for youthful looks?

In this book, you will learn about how to make the most out of getting older and how to reverse the negative effects of ageing. I also want to share with you all the tricks of the trade I have learnt in my long life and the secret to surviving in the best possible way, to enjoy life and feel younger than the date on your birth certificate.

Your biological age

I'm more than 20 years younger than my real age according to test results for biological age. Why? Because I have not accepted the traditional doomsday predictions of the ageing process. I have mentally told myself. Thank you, but no thank you. I will not go down that road to losing my identity as I get older.

I will teach you how-to reverse your biological age as well! It's not complicated, or expensive or very time consuming, but you have to use your mind as well as your body on a daily basis. Hopefully, you will love making an effort for your beautiful self. So, promise yourself you will feel happy about your age, accept the effects aging have on you, and work on everything that can reverse the negative and promote the positive.

Don't hide behind extra kilograms

I think it's sad to see women who have traded in their waistline for cakes and comfort foods and have given up the battle with the scales and calories by just adding on dangerous flabby fat. What is so sad is that all these overweight women are eating and relaxing themselves into hospitals, health problems and lots of unnecessary pain.

The great thing is that our bodies are extremely cooperative if we start the return-to-normal process. It will literally applaud you by quickly shedding fat and reducing inches. You will have healthier glowing skin and feel happier about yourself! Your mind will be lighter too, and you will gradually return to yourself as nature designed you!

Your life is worth the effort

It's far better to be a member of the club for women with a healthy lifestyle. That will be your insurance for a great life, good health and lasting good looks. When you look in the mirror and see that life is slowly slipping down to your ankles, don't be scared! You can do a lot to drag it back into place and become biologically younger, firmer, fitter and happier with your looks and your life. Will this take surgery, implants, expensive treatments and luxury products? Am I talking personal trainers and hours of daily work out, starving diets and hours of egocentric self-care?

Anti - ageing lifestyle

No, no, no!! I'm talking about a regime that can turn the clock back, improve your health, body and beauty all at a very low cost with a low maintenance level. You already have most of what you need for a New You around you in your own home and in your own body. It requires some effort, and at least 30 minutes a day. In this book, you will find all the advice and knowledge on being the best version of yourself, and the true key to rejuvenation and anti-ageing.

Everybody can afford it

It's much cheaper and easier than you think! It's absolutely true that you can use a lot from your kitchen cupboards to make super products for rejuvenation, skin and body care, health and increased energy.

The key to a New You is natural ingredients good enough to eat, for inner and outer transformation. Pamper your body with the best from nature, avoid as many manmade ingredients and preservatives as possible, and observe how your skin gradually becomes firmer, more glowing, younger and more radiant.

10 years younger

Combine your new and healthy beauty routines with improvements to your total lifestyle. Follow my eating and fitness plans on a daily basis. My best advice is that you make a plan, a schedule – and use 4 weeks to follow my New You plan.

Each week you will look and feel better! I can promise you that when your healthy New You month is over - you will feel and look fantastic. You will shed years – and literally become ten years younger. You will love what you see in the mirror. You will bubble with energy, confidence and happiness that you finally are on the right track to a healthy future!

Love your life and your looks

You will never be younger than you are right now At least not in years! But biologically you can become years younger if you make this effort for yourself. You can gain incredible results with simple changes, more than you can by spending a fortune on exclusive hype serums and creams. Lots of the glossy products are, sorry to say, snake oil...

I have been in the health and beauty business most of my long life, and I have tested and tried more or less everything worth mentioning. As owner and chief editor of the Norwegian leading lifestyle magazine Shape-Up, I have literally drowned in products, treatments and miracles. Lots of products are of course good, but my experience is "the more natural, the better".

Your fountain of youth

Our modern lifestyle has definite drawbacks with an overload of synthetic ingredients in foods, drinks and treatment products,and it's smart to be as restrictive as possible in order to avoid allergies and problems with your immune system.

In this post Corona times, we know how dangerous it is to be overweight, the main reason for the most common lifestyle diseases. To reduce the risk, the most important self-help treatment is to reduce your weight and waistline. You can do it quickly and efficiently by following the guidelines in this book. My combination of healthy eating/ menus and daily doses of simple exercises will improve your body far quicker than you can imagine. Extra bonus is far better general health and increased resistance to all kinds of health problems. It will make you stronger and less vulnerable to dangerous diseases as well as viruses and other germs.

Like I tell people when I have lifestyle lectures about my Eva method: The only thing you have to lose by following it – is fat and excess inches!

Creative cooking – Scandinavian Style

My cooking is based on a blending of Scandinavian and Mediterranean cooking, and it can easily be adjusted to your economy and what is available where you live. It is creative cooking, so you can add or subtract, change herbs and spices – and make them your own specialties. The idea is to bring joy to you cooking, as well as better health and looks.

I hope my book will inspire you to cook meals and to care for your skin in a delicious, healthy and rejuvenating way. I hope you will learn how to use your brain to influence your body on a cellular level, so it will react in a younger and healthier way day by day.

The fountain of youth is really bubbling inside you, and by transmitting the right signals from your brain to your body, you can really tap into it and enjoy all the benefits. I am sharing a lot of secrets with you to make you look younger and feel a lot better in every way. I promise you that the results will be awesome, and you will get a new kick out of life.

You will experience a surge of energy and optimism for the future, because you will realise that your age is not the important factor; it's how you look, how you feel, how you relate to the world around you.

I hope from the bottom of my heart that this book will be guide to your fountain of youth and joy!

All the best from Eva

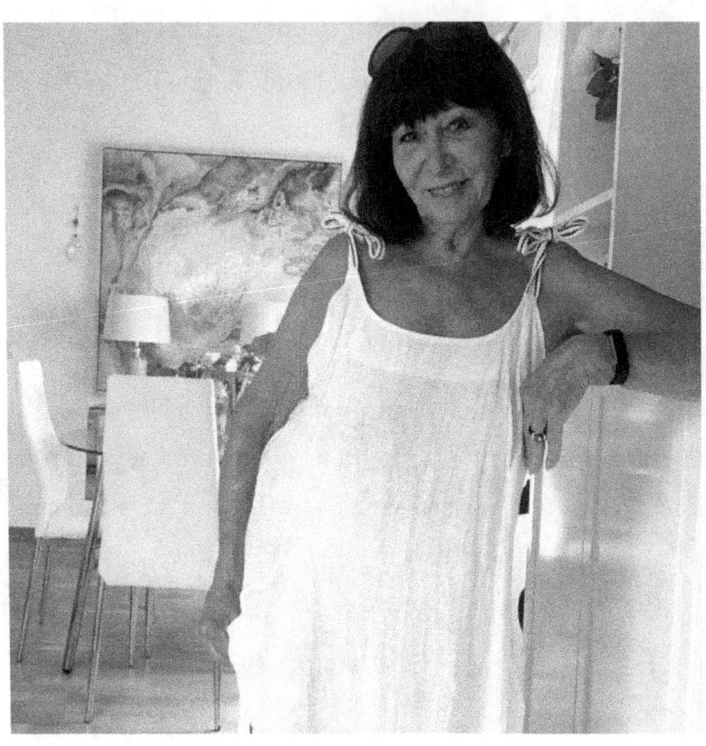

Chapter 2

YOUR NEW AND WONDERFUL LIFE

It's never too late to start a new life! It's never too late to renew and transform yourself into the person you really are. Do not just accept that age means getting old and frail, sick and helpless! Do not join the group of ageing people who are just waiting to become helpless and turn into mere shadows of themselves in the process. That is a dangerous and totally wrong attitude, whatever the experts say.

You are you!! All of your life

Advancing years does not mean that you have to be sliding downhill into lonely oblivion and decay. Aging does not mean that you are changing into a different person. You are you. A reflection of your genes, your background, environment - and your lifestyle, Inside, you are exactly the same person as you have always been.

A little wear and tear?

OK, so the exterior shows the imprints of life; laughter and sorrow lines, greying hair, love handles and sagging skin – too many wobbly extra pounds, and too little muscle... So what? This can be fixed to a large degree. You can restore yourself immensely if you are willing to make an effort for yourself.

You can reverse the ageing process, rejuvenate your looks, your way of thinking, acting and reacting! You can transform your mind, body, home and your surroundings.

It's in your power to make everything in your life fresh, new and exciting. Give it a chance for four short weeks and you will get a kick start to a New You!!

Are you worth it?

Do you think it sounds too tough for you? Or are you thinking this sounds great, but you will have to wait for results and that it's easier to relax and eat your good self into oblivion? This is NOT you!

Buying this book already means you are willing to invest some thoughts and elbow grease into your health, body and looks. That means you are really keen to make an effort to be a New and Healthier You.

Lifestyle is a free, green medicine

The good news is that you do not have to be a celebrity with loads of money to be the best version of yourself. No matter who you are and what kind of service you are able and willing to pay for, the main cost for transformation and maintenance is your daily effort. You can be a well-known celebrity, a multi-million-dollar heiress, or anybody, the daily effort is the same for us all. We all have to eat sensibly to reach (or maintain) the right weight for our height, frame and body type.

You have to do some strengthening exercises to regain muscle mass and reduce fat. You have to stretch to improve your flexibility and balance. You have to do some cardiovascular work in order to keep your oxygen level and circulatory system going, so your cells and organs will maintain nutrients and efficiently remove waste and toxins.

You have to use your brain, so it stays alert. You have to care for your skin to keep the largest organ of your body hydrated, nourished and elastic so it protects your internal organs. You have to think positive and look at the bright side of life and realize that you – and only you – can do the job!!

It's within reach for anybody, no matter what budget you are on. So really, it's like the Nike slogan: Just do it...

EVA'S TOP TEN TIPS

1. Maintain normal weight with healthy nutrition

2. Do strengthening exercises to keep muscle mass

3. Stretch to stay supple and flexible

4. Do cardio work and deep breathing for circulation

5. Use your brain by learning something new and challenging

6. Clean and care for your skin from top to toe

7. Get enough sleep

8. Think positive and have a proactive attitude

9. Meditate, visualize and brain train away your stress

10. Love, respect and honour yourself by taking super care of YOU

Many of you are probably already doing a lot of what I mention on this list. Others may not be. Whatever your current lifestyle, I'm pretty sure that this will give you the results you desire no matter what your starting point is. You will feel and look more youthful, increase your zest for life, and live your life better than ever! So, come on girls and decide that you are willing to do all it takes every day.

Invest a month of your life in You

Say YES, I am willing to do it and follow the NEW YOU system for a month! After these four weeks, you can decide whether this will be your permanent lifestyle or not. My bet is that you will continue! You will love your looks, you will love your boost of energy, and you will love getting older and better.

Are you still unsure? Are you hesitating to take the plunge into a new and more demanding life? Are you using excuses like, "I don't know exactly what to do, what I need, where and when to start"? Are you thinking, "It won't work for me because I'm too old, too fat, too out of shape. I have neglected myself for too long and nothing will really repair the wear and tear of my unhealthy, stressful life"?

You will succeed if you want to

I've heard all these excuses during my classes, my lectures and from thousands of women who have struggled to get out of a passive, fattening and ageing lifestyle into an active and rejuvenating one. And I have also heard their gratitude when they finally reach their normal weight and love themselves more. I have seen their pride and happiness when they realise they are the beautiful women they have always been.

Decide that you are worth the effort

So, no matter how long it takes to restore your beautiful you, get started today!! No more excuses because you are afraid of failing and disappointing yourself. Take it one day at a time. If you feel you haven't succeeded on one day, that's ok too. Just don't give up and start again the next day! Never blame yourself, just continue. Your new lifestyle is a permanent change, not a temporary diet or fitness fad. It's living for life.

It's living for a vibrant, healthy and beautiful you, no matter what age you are.

Transformation

This book is your guide to transforming yourself into a New You, or rather retrieving the vibrant You buried inside a lifetime of living. Maybe you have been too busy with your work, your family and your daily life to focus on yourself and your personal needs. Like most of us, you have probably postponed the better eating habits, the fitness program, the beauty regime until next Monday.

Then you (like the rest of us) suddenly realise that years of Mondays have passed, and you have paid little attention to your own body, soul and well-being.

But there is still to renew and restore what we have neglected so you will get a lot of mileage on the highway of the rest of your life. And the best thing is you will thoroughly enjoy the trip! I can guarantee you that if you invest one month – four weeks/ 120 days of your life focusing on your own transformation, you will get hooked on this fabulous new lifestyle of yours for the rest of your life. You will feel on top of the world and wonder why you never did it before.

It's never ever too late, so let's get started!!

Chapter 3

YOUR NEW YOU PLAN

Like in business and projects, we always start with a plan, a budget and a schedule. This project is "NEW YOU" and the product is you. I have put together my experiences and knowledge of nutrition, fitness, preventive health, beauty, styling, relaxation and motivation techniques in this condensed and effective plan that is easy to follow.

1. Easy, no matter what your starting point is

2. Affordable, no matter what your budget is

3. Enjoyable, no matter what your interests/abilities are

4. Goal oriented, effective and within reach in a short time

I hope I can inspire and coach you to make it really fun to renew yourself and your life. I sincerely hope from my heart of hearts that this book will be your source of inspiration, and your companion to becoming the New You for the rest of your wonderful life.

Your wonderful body

You will probably disagree with me when I say you have a wonderful body. Most women look in the mirror and dislike or hate what they see. All they may perceive is a protruding stomach, sagging breasts, flabby thighs, a wobbly bum, cellulite and ageing skin: the tell-tale signs of a life lived and, honestly, too much food, too little exercise, plus not spending enough time on self-care.

Like most of us, you probably get depressed by the look of things and you feel it's a hopeless task to return your body to its former glory. It's not!! Of course, let's be sensible – you will never be sweet sixteen again (and thank heavens for that), but you can get most of your body parts back where they belong if you work at it. If things have slipped slowly down to your ankles, get a grip on the cover that is you and drag it up again. You can do this.

Step by step

No matter what shape or form you are in just now, I can promise you that each week from now on you will get more of yourself back. If you follow the daily routine, you will like what you see in the mirror in one short month.

And each month from now – for the rest of your life – you will see more and more improvement instead of more and more 'decay'. So, it's up to you, baby! Read on. It's important that you have all the information first, do some thinking, and then take some action.

Food, glorious food

Food can be your best friend, or your worst enemy. The right foods in the right quantity prepared the right way are the best health and beauty source on this planet. The wrong foods in the wrong quantities can be sheer poison and ruin your health, your looks, and your well-being. Nutrition-depleted industrial foods combined with the stress and requirements of our modern society, a lack of exercise, fresh air, and manual labour will all contribute to rapid ageing and health problems.

Dangerous obesity

One of the main health problems of the Western world is obesity and the rapidly increasing number of overweight people. It's not only the extra pounds, but the fact that this extra weight is sheer fat and flab. This larder is only meant to be a temporary survival source of calories in times of hunger, and it's still extremely important in countries where food is scarce, and people are solely dependent on their crop yields.

In the Western world, this ability to store food has turned into one of our major health threats. Food is available in abundance, everywhere, at all times.

Unfortunately, many foods and drinks are loaded with fats, sugars, refined carbohydrates, additives, artificial tastes and colours, and they are very low in nutritional value. Much of it can also be downright dangerous for your health!

Smarter choices for health and beauty

Fortunately, you have a choice! You can go for real natural produce available in many stores. You just have to be selective and choose good nutrition and good taste for your money.

Think quality not quantity.

It's smart to avoid processed food with glossy pictures and start buying the real thing in natural packaging. Touch, smell, evaluate, and choose the best produce you can for your money, your body, and your looks. The right foods are the energy your cells need to function properly, and they deserve the real thing, not synthetic crap.

The natural way

Hippocrates said, "Your food is your medicine, your medicine is your food." He also said, "Give me fever, and I can cure all diseases." It's strange that all doctors still pledge the Hippocratic Oath when they are certified, but few Western doctors are using the know-how of this ancient healer.

Unfortunately, modern medicine is based on relatively new pharmaceutical products, aimed at destroying invaders of the body more than supporting and strengthening its own immense healing powers.

In my opinion, most illnesses are the manifestations of imbalances in the cells and the normal functions of body (or brain) often related to severe stress, pollution, and damaging lifestyles. Illnesses occur when the immune system is overtaxed and cannot cope with invaders anymore. It starts to deteriorate, and the cry for help is effectively silenced by medicines.

You can create lifelong diseases

Unfortunately, most medicines have side effects, and you need other medicines (with other side effects) to treat or silence the original side effects. Before you know it, you are a VIP customer at the pharmacy.

This is not the fault of the doctors; most are doing a great job, but it's (again in my opinion) the education and brainwashing they have received through Big Pharma throughout their studies.

Nowadays, the internet is gradually improving the medical know- how of consumers, so you can make better choices. It's smart if you think and act more in line with the philosophy and know-how of Hippocrates: Your food is your medicine; your medicine is your food!!

Help your body to heal itself and help it function better on a daily basis. Find a doctor who understands the value of nutrition, lifestyle, and the mind-body connection, who can guide you, support you and sees you like a human being, not only as a source of income!

Your normal weight

Wallis Simpson, the Duchess of Windsor, once said you can never be too skinny, or too rich. Unfortunately, this has had a big impact on Western women. I think it's really scary to see all the anorexic, starved and super skinny models and celebrities that are our modern-day icons.

It's actually slightly crazy that women are starving themselves and look like ten-year-old boys, then add on big breast implants and cosmetic surgery.

I much prefer the Italian saying: After 40, you have to choose between your face and your bum... Don't despair if you are above the fashionable starvation level. Let's focus on you and your looks and how to feel really good about yourself. Let's see what can be done with what nature has given you.

Analyse your body

It's truth time! Even if you hate the scales, you have to step on them to get a realistic starting point. At the end of this book you will find charts to fill in to keep track of your progress. This is an extremely important section, as it will show you exactly where you are on your way to a New You during the process.

Remember, it's for your eyes only, and it's time to be very honest with yourself. This will make you stick to your program, and not hide your head in the sand any longer. Face facts and make a serious effort for the New You. Four weeks from now, you will see the amazing results, and your weight and measurements will be reduced more than you imagine!

Your self confidence and self image will increase accordingly, and you will love smiling back at your gorgeous reflection in the mirror. You have nothing else to lose except worthless flab.

Ten pounds at the time

When you follow this eating plan you will lose fat – the ugly yellow, greasy stuff that is harmful to your body, your organs and your blood.

The eating plan will give you enough food to keep you feeling full and it's packed with great nutrients and energy to boost your metabolism and well-being. It might be different from what you are eating now (what made you overweight in the first place) and it might take a bit of time to get used to new eating habits, but please, please follow the plan.

Aim for a weight loss of two to three pounds a week, which means you will lose a minimum of 10 pounds in a month. The more overweight you are, the more you will lose.

Remember that you will also be doing the fitness program that builds muscle mass at the same time, so the actual loss of fat will be substantially higher. You will see it in how your clothes fit and you will rapidly drop in sizes. To register the inch loss, you will use a measuring tape for figure control every week and fill in the body control form at the end of the book.

Size down, motivation up

Seeing your measurements shrink is motivation number one. The flabbier you are, the faster your fitness program will reduce your measurements. I know what I'm talking about, and I can assure you that this is not an empty promise.

During my long career as one of the leading health, beauty, and lifestyle experts in Norway, I have helped thousands of Norwegian women of all age groups with my system through a coast-to-coast network of slimming and fitness instructors.

Amazing makeovers with a new lifestyle

The women who have followed my system have gained better bodies, better health, and better lifestyles. Many have been featured in leading Norwegian magazines, as they have totally transformed their bodies and their lives for the better.

Your own reality story

I do recommend you keep your own diary during the process, as it's very motivating and helpful in order to stay on the straight and narrow. You can also make your own videos and share your feelings, challenges, results etc. with yourself, just like on a reality TV series.

If you are brave enough, you can share your story on Facebook or other social media; this is a fantastic way to keep you on the road to success. It will surely also inspire others, and it might give you lots of positive input.

Selfies

If you ask someone to take pictures of you along the way, it will also be a great tool on your route to rejuvenation. Take pictures from the front, the side, and the back in the same underwear and with the same light each time. You won't believe your own eyes after a month, and you will see your gradual transformation. If you are you afraid of showing your body to someone else, you can try to take the photos yourself using a mirror as this will be of great importance on your road to success!

Love your body with your brain

It's the only one you have got! It's very, very important that you get friendly with your body. It's so very precious, because it's your very own vehicle on this planet during this life. If you hate it, your brain will surely respond accordingly. It will protest, it will feel neglected and unloved, and it will respond to your negative attitude by living up to the signals you send to it.

Thoughts manifest themselves in reality

It's a well-known fact that the mind-body connection is extremely important, and that the body responds to the images sent by the conscious and unconscious parts of your brain. It's an intricate biological feedback system that is highly influenced by your thoughts. Send the signal fat, ugly, old, etc., and the obedient brain transfers response signals to make the image a reality. Send the signal cellulite and the dreaded orange peel skin will manifest.

Try to alter the signals, your body image, your feelings regarding your body and your whole self! Start with positive affirmations, which are a kind of personal brain wash, and you will gradually alter your way of thinking in an amazing way and you will feel much better about your body and your whole person.

Be nice to your body. Be your own best friend and life coach. Embrace your whole self and do the best you can along the way.

Never give up – be a winner

If you fail for a day or two, so what? It's not the end of the world! It will just take you a few days longer to achieve the results you want. Remember, we are not talking about a limited period of just another diet.

We are talking about a whole, long-lasting life and body transformation based on permanent change and an improvement in your total lifestyle and way of thinking and acting. Only this permanent change in your thoughts and feelings can change your looks, your health, reverse the ageing process, and reduce your biological age for the rest of your life.

We are talking feeling good forever!

We are boosting our quality of life as long as it lasts. I have written a lot of different affirmations for you later in this book, and I recommend that you repeat them as often as possible like a mantra. The more you use them, the more they will work for you by transforming your dreams into realities.

<h1 style="text-align:center">Chapter 4</h1>

THE SECRETS OF A NEW YOU

Amazing improvements are possible without liposuction, starvation diets, and personal trainers. You can be your own body expert by following the step-by-step instructions in this book. Everything you do is for your own well-being, your own looks, your own zest for life, and your own future!

Each week from now on you will be happier with your reflection and the way you feel about yourself and your life. You will prove that you can do it, that you are worth the effort. You will know for sure that it's within your power, and yours alone, to create your extreme make-over and make you a New You! The real you....

Let's start with some basic facts that make the whole process more logical and will give you the incentive to relate everything to your unique biochemical identity.

Realise that we are all different, that some people can load down calories 24/7, and still be slim and even have flat tummies without ever doing a sit up. Stop envying them. You are different, so accept who you are and know what your unique body needs to stay slim and healthy.

Don´t even try to copy your skinny friends with high metabolisms; we all have insecurities and they are no different. So, get the basic know how about how YOU can stay within your perfect metabolic range.

The energy balance

You probably know that 1 kg of pure fat (no water) represents 9,000 kcal. This is what you will find stated on food packaging. This kind of fat is more concentrated than body fat because your body contains more water.

On average, 1 kg of body fat represents approximately 7,000 kcal of energy (2000 less than pure food fat). Simple arithmetic shows that to lose 1 kg of body fat you must reduce your intake of calories by the same amount.

An even better alternative is to increase your activity level and burn off 7,000 kcal, but this is tough unless you are a serious athlete, which presumably you are not since you want to change your body weight and shape.

The realistic and far better option is to combine a reduction of your intake of calories in foods and drinks and burn off more by increasing your activity level and building more muscle mass. My system is all about this sensible and healthy combination.

Increase your metabolism

Activity has a lot of other positive effects on your body, both inside and outside. When you exercise intensively for a minimum of 30 minutes, your resting metabolism will increase by approximately 15%. This means that you will automatically burn 15% more calories than you normally do. This is almost the same increase seen with medication to treat low thyroid function and low metabolism.

The amazing added benefit is that this effect will be sustained for the 12 hours after just 30 minutes of exercise. If you really want very quick results for fat loss and body reshaping, motivate yourself to work out morning and evening, and your metabolism will work at full speed 24/7.

This is the key for anybody with a sluggish metabolism, and far better than using prescription medications to normalise it (unless it is seriously low).

Has slimming made you fat?

Many women have a sluggish metabolism because they have experimented with so many diets during their life. This has caused a gradual reduction in their resting metabolism and their fat burning capacity. This is the survival response of the body when it's getting too little food. It puts on all the brakes to save your body from starvation.

Lowering the metabolism is actually an important survival technique for humans, particularly as it's combined with an increased capacity to store energy as body fat to save lives when food is scarce. Modern starvation is usually in the form of self induced, calorie-restricted diets, but your body and brain do not know the difference.

The signals of danger and starvation increase the ability to store fat in exactly the same way the body responds to famine.

The signals are danger, danger: slow down metabolism, increase fat storage functions, lower energy levels, decrease fat-burning capacity, lower resting metabolism" etc. The sorry result is that you can lose five pounds by more or less starving yourself on an unbalanced, low- nutrition dense diet and then put it back on or gain more.

YoYo syndrome

After you have lost weight by starving yourself, you start eating a little bit more, but very sensibly. Then you notice you've put on the lost pounds as quick as a flash, and also some extra pounds: The diet actually made you fatter.

No, it's a struggle to lose even more pounds, and the vicious health hazard cycle becomes a long-term lifestyle fact.

You have started an uphill struggle: dieting yourself into a gradually increasing weight problem. If you are one of the many, many women who have ended up in this cycle, here you will learn how to break it and you can get back on the healthy path.

Back to normal

To kick your metabolism back to normal requires that you combine food and supplements. It might take time as well as effort, but what's the alternative? Eating like a bird and getting as fat as a pig?

Take a month of your life to shape up your metabolism again. By gradually increasing your activity level and adjusting your eating habits, you will be able to eat more while still losing fat, gaining much more energy and far better health.

Increased activity will also normalize the automatic regulation of your appetite: the energy balancing system of the body. When your system functions normally, it makes it very easy to maintain normal body weight without weighing and measuring, counting calories, carbs, fats or being focused on "slimming". The body will regulate hunger and satiety automatically when it's treated right and gets the minimum amount   of movement each day. Follow my food plan and step on the scales each morning to see how much you lose.

EXTRA BONUS FOR YOU

1. Improved circulation of oxygen-rich blood to all cells

2. Clearer complexion, glowing skin tone

3. Firmer, more elastic skin all over

4. Shapely body with more defined shape

5. Stronger, younger body, better balance and posture

6. Improved digestion, less harmful toxins in your body

7. Increased oxygen intake and improved breathing

8. Decrease in negative stress

9. Better sleep

10. Quicker thinking and mental alertness

11. Increased production of endorphins, the feel-good hormones of your body

12. Boosted immune system

13. Improved bodily functions

Chapter 5

FIGHT SELF SABOTAGE

How to get started

It's a great challenge to say farewell to old habits and introduce (and stick to) new ones. Very often we know what to do, and how to do it, but we keep postponing until next Monday. We find a lot of excuses to put it of for just another day, and for many people this ends with never.

It's very important that you are honest with yourself and that you decide to outsmart your inner saboteur. This little monster tries to get you to be (or keep you) a wobbly, ageing, lazy person.

Stop listening to this sweet talk with all the excuses for just relaxing. Relaxing can mean the end of the healthy, attractive person you want to be. Your little inner monster hates change and has a long list of reasons for you to stay the same, relax and put of healthy eating, working out, and personal care.

Tomorrow is another day
and tomorrow and tomorrow

I can write pages with more depressing arguments from the little subconscious monster inside you. How can you outsmart and silence it? By literally knocking it out and sending these thoughts into oblivion. Or perhaps it's an even better idea to brainwash it with positive healthy thoughts so these messages cooperate on your road to a New You.

Let's have a look at the sweet talk from the slimming saboteur monster.....

1. You are tired and you need to relax

2. You can start your fitness program on Monday

3. You can start your diet tomorrow

4. You need a lot of preparation to get started

5. You must watch your favourite TV programs

6. You deserve to relax with a good book

7. You must phone your friends

8. You must surf the net

9. You must check in with your Facebook friends

10. The weather is too cold, too wet, or too hot

11. There is no space for a workout in your home

12. You need fitness equipment

13. You need comfort food, a drink, some chocolate, a slice of cake

14. You are lonely and you need to feel sorry for yourself

15. Nobody cares about how you look anyway

16. You are too old, so you deserve to pamper yourself with food, drinks
    and the easy life

17. You will not succeed anyway

18. You do not have the willpower to get started

19. Exercise will be diffcult with your stiff joints

20. You will feel so clumsy and hopeless, so why even start?

A list of great answers to get out of your comfort zone:

1. *I am tired because I´m out of shape. I need to get my bum into action, out of the sofa*

2. *I need to get started now, not on Monday! I will start this very minute*

3. *I have eggs, salad, and water! I can start my healthy eating diet today*

4. *I will plan and prepare and act today*

5. *I can do sit-ups when I watch TV*

6. *I can read and relax in bed when I have finished my NEW YOU program*

7. *I can chat with friends later - or another day*

8. *I can surf the net when I have my morning coffee*

9. *I can check Facebook after my workout*

10. *I can dress for any kind of weather*

11. *There is plenty of space for my yoga mat and myself*

12. *All I need is my own body*

13. *I need healthy foods that make me feel and look good, So I do not need comfort foods that stay five minutes in my mouth and the rest of my life around my waist*

14. *I am not lonely anymore because I have started on a new and positive lifestyle with plenty to do. I do not feel sorry for myself any longer because I am in control of my own body and my own future. It will give me a lot of new life opportunities*

15. *I'm doing this because I care about myself and this will influence how I act with other people and I certainly think they will care too*

16. *I am not too old! I will reverse the whole ageing process so my biological age will be years younger than my birth age*

17. *I can do it. I will do it because I have decided to be a winner*

18. *I will succeed by being goal oriented, and I will be using my willpower, my brain and my body every day from now on*

19. *My muscles are stiff from lack of exercise, so I will stretch them softly back to flexibility and strength and build stronger muscles to protect and support my body*

20. *Nobody will see how clumsy I am now, as I work out alone with no audience. I am certainly not a hopeless case. I will improve day by day, and gradually get fit*

Tell yourself

- *Tomorrow is another day! Each tomorrow, I will be better, healthier and happier*

- *I will enjoy life to the fullest*

- *I will enjoy my new eating habits*

- *I will get the great satisfaction of being a winner, proving to myself that I can do it*

- *I will love my NEW me*

Chapter 6

YOUR BODY CONTROL

Get feedback in black and white. "The New You Body Control Chart" is a valuable tool to keep you on the straight and narrow, and it will be extremely motivating to see the gradual improvements of your body. I recommend that you fill it in twice a week.

To get the numbers right you need an ordinary tape measure and scales. You need to see yourself naked. Hating what you see in the mirror and on the scales is like hiding your head in the sand. It's better to face facts and get a clear picture of what you are working with to find out what need's improvement.

Instant inch loss

Stand relaxed and take all the measurements of your naked body. Jot the figures down on the form. Then pull in your stomach and note down the measurement. Do the same with your butt, arms, etc., and see how many inches you lose just by pulling in your muscles.

When you follow the fitness program every day, you see inch loss in these measurements even if you don't lose weight on the scales. By firming up, you can easily drop a dress size and look a lot better because your whole body will be more toned.

Fill in the form with your new measurements every week from now on, on the same day of the week, to keep track of your progress.

I can promise you that you will see amazing improvements in a very short time. Before you know it, you will get your own firm and shapely body back.

One day at a time

If you have a lot of extra kilograms (or stones) to lose, it will of course take time, but you will be slimmer and firmer every week from now on if you stick to the system.

The heavier you are, the more you lose to start with because you will lose a lot of water weight. On average, you can lose up to 1 kg of body fat each week with your new lifestyle.

To visualise this, take four packs of 250 g butter, which is a little less than 1 kg body fat.

Imagine what getting rid of four packs of buttery fat each week from your body will mean for your size, your looks, and your wellness. You will be on the way to a fabulous New You, feeling and looking better each week from now on.

Know your body type

We are all different, and this is fantastic. Imagine how boring the world would be if we all looked like long-legged, super slim, beautiful models. If we are not careful, we could be on our way to a very unhealthy attitude towards looks. In the last few years, thankfully there have been gradually more and more models that look like us.

Unhealthy role models

The trendsetters are celebrities. Most celebrities are scared to get older, to look older, and they pay whatever it takes in money and pain to stop time. Many still look old, but in a totally strange way. This is evident with before and after shots of the rich and famous with shiny, stretched, pink or dead-pale skin (thanks to chemical peeling) or immobilised features (thanks to Botox). Combined with new, regular, big and stop-traffc white teeth, they can look downright scary.

Sensible cosmetic surgery

I do understand, of course, that plastic surgery, peelings and fillers can bring new confidence for those who have a problem that bothers them daily, like oversized features, acne-scarred skin, bags under the eyes and heavy lids.

Some women with smaller busts feel that implants are the only solution for them to look and feel more feminine. This is very understandable! Some women can also suffer from large breasts and related health problems, and they need breast reduction to improve their quality of life.

Often though, women with larger breasts are also overweight and unfit and should get down to normal weight before opting for the trauma of surgery to get the best and healthiest result. The same goes for all kinds of liposuction, breast implants, tummy tucks, and tightening of flabby upper arms and thighs.

Images in celebrity magazines are perfected in Photoshop so no scars are visible. Very few talk about the pain, the risks or the dangerous side effects of these surgeries, but they assure you they are major surgical procedures in the name of beauty and eternal youth. Don´t be fooled!!

Your shape and body type

All body types are attractive when they are normal weight and have enough muscles to keep them firm. However, when lots of fat is accumulated and muscle mass is lost, the ratio between fat and lean body mass is altered and it's an entirely different matter.

The beautiful body shape is hidden behind layers of fat and this radically alters the look of your body. Here are the main body types:

Hourglass

This has always been considered the perfect feminine body. Bust and hip measurements are more or less the same, and the waist is approximately 10 inches smaller. It's a harmonious body with nice proportions, but when it gets fatter it becomes more voluptuous.

Triangle

This body type is often tall, with long legs, narrow hips, broader shoulders and big breasts. The waist is not well defined. When a woman with a triangle body gains weight, the fat deposits are on the upper torso. Gradually they become very top heavy, and they get potbellies and a bigger bust.

This masculine-type fat storage is dangerous and can easily lead to diabetes and cardiovascular diseases. It can also cause neck and back trouble as the heavy bust is a constant strain on the body and creates an imbalance in posture.

Pear

This is the feminine mother earth goddess body! Often the shoulders are narrow and sloping and breasts are small to medium. The waist is narrow when the body weight is normal. The hips are wider, the thighs and often the legs are heavier.

Cellulite is very common as circulation tends to be sluggish. Extra weight usually shows up on the lower body. When slimming/ dieting without working out, weight is often lost on the upper body and chest.

Square

This type of body is heavy and strong. The shoulders are straight and often broad, and the breasts are small to medium. These women tend to have a flat stomach and bum, not very defined waist - and medium, but often muscular, thighs and legs.

If a woman with a square body puts on weight, it's evenly distributed all over. They can put on quite a lot before it's noticeable, but when they cross the line to fat, these bodies can look more masculine.

Rectangular

This is a taller and often naturally slimmer body. Actually, quite a number of models have this body type. It can be rather androgynous and is often stiff and needs stretching. If they put on weight, it's often all over the body.

Apple

This is a body with a bigger bust, protruding stomach and lack of waist, often combined with slimmer thighs and legs, flat bum and thinner arms.

Lots of body types turn to apples as they grow older. It's partly hormonal, but it's also related to obesity and inactivity. It's unhealthy fat distribution that can lead to a multitude of lifestyle diseases.

Whatever shape your body is, please accept it, love it, and make the best of it. When you reach normal weight and have a good ratio between fat and muscle tissue, you will look great regardless!

Chapter 7

FLYING START WITH DETOX

If you have read my book, The Green Lifestyle Detox Diet, you will know most of the content in this chapter, but it's important to remind yourself and it's a must for new readers. This is, in my opinion, the key to renewing and restoring your health and your looks.

A healthy body gives a healthy soul: Corpore mens sana corpore est (a healthy mind in a healthy body).

Let's take a good look inside your body, starting with your complex plumbing system. Detox is all about cleaning and scrubbing out all the garbage in your system.

Your body is not a garbage can

Get rid of all the food that will no longer be part of your life. The first step to a cleaner, healthier body is to have a critical eye for all the contents of your kitchen cupboards, your fridge, and freezer.

Perhaps these need a good clearing out to get rid of the stuff that isn't good for you. Say goodbye to foods and drinks that are loaded with empty, unhealthy carbs, bad fats, sugar, sweeteners and other additives. They belong in the garbage can not in (or on) your body!

Stay clear of this type of food for at least one month, and I can promise you that you will never return to them on a daily basis when you notice how you feel and look.

In my system, nothing is totally forbidden! You are not going to turn into a boring food fanatic! You are going to enjoy food and life to the fullest. Of course, you can have a taste of everything you desire, but only once in a while as a special treat.

Declutter and get rid of unhealthy food

If you have a lot of other fattening foods that are not good for you in your kitchen, you should get rid of it all now. Clear out, wash and reorganize! When you have done some major clearing, the next thing is to fill up the shelves, the fridge, the freezer with the New You foods.

If you are a chocolate or sugar addict, it will take a while for your body to quit the craving. Why? Hormones. Chocolate is real comfort and feel-good food because it releases endorphins – the natural opiates of the body that make you slightly high – and numbs pain.

Try to compensate with other ways of raising your endorphin levels. Jogging, work outs, and sex are great alternatives!

Your blood sugar

If you are used to monosaccharides – refined sugars that immediately heighten your blood sugar level – you need to stop eating any kind of white sugar and white flour. Both are disastrous for our health and rocket our risk of diabetes. It's extremely taxing on our systems, which have to produce insulin in much higher doses than they are designed to.

An inside look

Your colon is five feet long and is coiled to fit inside your relatively small body. This means there are a lot of places where food particles can easily get stuck. Imagine a colon so full of old "leftovers" that it slowly and constantly releases toxins that travel around your body.

The toxic environment will naturally influence your cells. They protect themselves, which can gradually alter their natural functions. This will influence all your organs.

The result is that you feel tired, you feel negative and out of shape, you have trouble sleeping, and you have more stiffness, aches and pains than normal. Other toxic signals are that you feel bloated, constipated, and have very irregular bowel movements. Your skin and hair will lose shine and elasticity.

Detox is a must to get your insides sparkling clean and to give you and your body a healthy new start.

Firm up your colon

Most people gradually get small pockets (diverticulitis) in their colon when they get older. These slack pockets are weaknesses in the colon tissue that is supposed to be elastic and firm. When it's slack and has pockets, more fermented garbage will become stuck there and more and more toxins are created.

Your immune defense system will be working overtime to save you from toxic damage, meaning it has far less time and resources to fight other invaders, and this means you are much more sensitive to all kinds of infections and diseases.

When I lecture on this subject, I always give this example: Leave a pork chop in the same nice and warm environment as your colon for a week or two and imagine the smell, the rot, the poison.

Not to scare you, but it gives you an idea of why it's really smart to start your new lifestyle with a serious detox. This example works, as my students get on the Detox Diet quicker than you can say the phrase.

Roughage is important

It's easier than you think to follow my Detox Diet because you can chew and eat, not only drink. I have never been a fan of total fasting or only fluids because this tends to lower your resting metabolism. This can backfire and cause you to gain weight after fasting. It can also lead to less muscle mass, as the body uses protein in the muscles for repairs and new growth.

In my experience, detoxing with lots of roughage combined with lots of fluids will scrub and cleanse the colon. To make this even more efficient, include a little vegetable oil to lubricate the lining and make everything slip trough more easily.

This combination is extremely potent and efficient for every person suffering from constipation or a lazy colon due to overuse of laxatives and/ or a lack of exercise and lack of roughage in their daily diet.

My advice: If you have a lazy colon issue, it's important that you take a Detox Day at least once a week to be sure that you get rid of all toxins before they accumulate and become dangerous to your health and well-being.

New You Detox Program

Detox is about total cleansing of your body, inside and outside. This means a combination of eating, drinking, moving, washing, scrubbing and sweating and I recommend three days of purification to start with.

It's smart if you can be totally focused on the Detox plan; it's a healthy ego trip that will allow your body to enter rejuvenation mode.

Many prefer to take a weekend in solitude and get a kick start on their new life. That's great if you have the opportunity, but if not, plan how you can incorporate the plan in your normal program carefully.

Morning

When you wake up, stretch like a cat! Tell yourself that this will be a glorious and magical day! Tell yourself that this is a day to take super care of yourself and your precious body! Convince yourself that you are on the right track to a fabulous and healthy body and better looks.

Tell yourself that you certainly will enjoy your new lifestyle more than your old one! Get out of bed, put on your robe, and start cleaning up.

- First take one teaspoonful of best quality cold-pressed virgin olive oil.

- Then drink four to six glasses of lukewarm, still mineral water. You can add the juice of half a lemon to fortify it.

- Brush and floss your teeth and tongue. Splash tepid, then cold water on your face to give it a wakeup call.

- Put on a comfortable workout outfit. Roll out your yoga mat.

- Put on relaxing music, and good morning to you! If it's not too cold outside, open the windows and let the fresh air in.

Deep breathing detox exercises

Inhale as much air as possible, hold for five seconds, and exhale slowly. Repeat 10 times and increase daily up to 20 or more. Switch on your best workout music.

Workout and get energised

I recommend that you get your metabolism going at full speed by doing the complete New You workout for 30 minutes minimum. The alternative is to put on music and walk at a brisk pace around the house. Skip, jump, stretch, dance, move your arms, and get really sweaty. You can find a lot of great walking videos on YouTube.

Whatever you choose, it's so important to get your metabolism going, so keep your heart rate up and sweat for at least 20 minutes so your body burns fat, not only glucose.

This is how you can increase your resting metabolism for 12 hours after a 30-minute hard workout. If you work out twice a day, you will benefit from significantly higher burning of fat 24/7. I can promise you that you will see the fantastic results of your efforts, so fantastic that you gradually will love your workouts!

Detox your skin

Then cleanse your face. Use a face brush in circular movements to stimulate cell rejuvenation and polish your skin. You can also "dust" of your skin with a stiff face cloth (or linen napkin) in circular movements until the skin is red and warm.

Then it's time for serious dry brushing to renew the skin of your whole body. Use exfoliating gloves or a long-handled brush all over. It's a very efficient and natural way to remove dead skin cells while also increasing your circulation to detox your skin. It will also clear the pores, so they are ready to absorb the ingredients in your natural massage oil: olive oil with drops of essential oils like Rosemary, Ylang-Ylang, or other oils that you like.

Self massage

Massage from toe to top slowly, following the lymphatic system. Massage your face and neck gently. Massage oil into your scalp and press the points on your cranium to increase energy.

Massage extra moisturizer into your face and neck and leave it on like a cream mask. Put a shower cap on your head and wrap a towel around it so the heat increases, and the oils can penetrate your hair.

Have your breakfast and give the oils and creams time to be absorbed into your skin and hair before you shower and shampoo.

Chapter 8

EVA'S DETOX DIET

Detox Breakfast

Drink as many cups of herbal tea as possible and make extra tea to keep in bottles for drinking during the day. Lemon, ginger, mint, chai and dandelion are good choices.

Prepare Detox juice

Cut up two apples, one carrot, a celery stick, half a cucumber, quarter of a lemon, and mint leaves and have it all in a juicer.

Blend with two cups of mineral water. Drink one cup and save the rest for the evening. If you don´t have a juicer, you make an extra-large portion of the raw food salad.

Enjoy a big portion of raw food

Cut an apple, carrot and celery sticks into small cubes or grate with grated lemon peel on top. Add a teaspoon of olive oil and a little apple cider vinegar or lemon juice and a touch of salt as dressing.

Detox Supplements

Milk Thistle, Organic Spirulina, different algae powders and/ or green clay are all great for naturally cleansing your liver and other internal organs. They will also improve your immune defence system.

Shower and Change

Time to get the oil of (if there is any left on your skin and in your hair). Use a little bit of shower gel on a big, fluffy sponge and massage your body, following the lymphatic pathways. Shampoo and condition your hair.

Dry with a coarse terry towel and then massage lots of body lotion all over. Moisturize your face and neck and slap your face to get the glowing skin tone back. Put on light makeup, blow dry and style your hair, and get dressed for the day.

Enjoy the ego trip

This week is all about you, your well-being, and your rejuvenation, so allow yourself to be totally selfish and just focus on improving yourself until it becomes part of your daily routine. Don't let your partner or anyone else distract you from your "me time".

Relax and meditate

Relax and do some deep breathing after breakfast and repeat the following affrmations:

I am (your name) here and now.

I am healthy, happy, young and beautiful.

I love my body, I love my life.

I am saying goodbye to the past.

I welcome my wonderful future!

Please do not change these affirmations. Just say them over and over and over again like a mantra. This will reprogram your subconscious mind and gradually make your affirmations come to life. This is really the universal key to happiness and the secret behind my New You system!

I hope from the bottom of my heart that you will take the time to use the system so it gradually will become a wonderful part of your happy, healthy life.

I am convinced that if you do, the system will help you to shape up your body and brain, renew you, and bring harmony and happiness to you for the rest of your life.

Detox lunch

Drink a quarter of a cup of pure Aloe Vera Barbadensis juice to restore your intestines on a cellular level. It's optional, but I recommend it if you really want total inside-out restoration. Enjoy your healthy Aloe Vera drink while you mix a big bowl of colourful salad.

Detox salad

Choose a mixture of carrots, oranges, ginger, parsley, garlic, beets, celery, parsnips, apples, onions and sweet peppers – all or some, as you like. You can add grains of wheat, oats, barley or some sprouts for extra taste, crunch and lots of extra vitamins and minerals.

Make a dressing from olive oil, fresh lemon juice, a touch of salt, black pepper, and chopped garlic. You can even add extra herbs if you like.

Drink a lot to flush out toxins

Drink lots of water with slices of lemon or cucumber. Drink detoxifying dandelion, cinnamon, lemon, or chamomile tea. These are also tasty with crushed ice or ice cubes served in tall glasses with slices of lemon and a few cherries.

If you need sweetener, use Stevia – it is a natural herb that tastes sweeter than sugar. Get used to it, and save lots of calories in a healthy, green way.

Rest and relax

After lunch, just relax and meditate lying at on the floor on your back while concentrating on deep cleansing breathing. Gradually you can practice your affirmations to cleanse your thoughts. Between meals, don't eat or drink anything, except as much water as you can drink. The more you drink, the more it will help your kidneys to cleanse out your whole system.

Afternoon walk

Your feet are made for walking, and rejuvenating oxygen is free for all. So, get out in the fresh air and enjoy the world around you. It's so good for you. If you have followed the program, you already look pretty good with glossy, clean hair, some light makeup, and with glowing skin from your morning workout and skincare routine.

Check the weather and dress accordingly. Dress sporty or casual, but style yourself so you like what you see in the mirror. Today you want to feel good and look your best. Of course, avoid the old, saggy, baggy trousers and the tatty tracksuit. Those outfits belong in the garbage can, not on the New You.

Look good, feel great

My best advice is to wear something that would make you feel good if you were meeting someone you had a crush on years ago. Bring a water bottle to be sure you are hydrated and walk at a brisk pace.

Feel how your muscles work when you try different movements with your arms and legs. It's all about getting to know you and that precious body of yours.

Detox afternoon snack

When you get home, I bet you will feel really good about yourself and the new physical you. Enjoy the feeling! Drink lots and lots of water or herbal tea while you prepare this super healthy afternoon treat.

Vegetarian snack paste

Chop four cloves of garlic and mix with one tablespoon of olive oil. Add finely chopped parsley and bay laurel (optional) to the paste before serving. Spread it on small squares of whole grain or crisp bread.

If you prepare bigger portions and keep it in a glass jar in the fridge, you will have a great paste for pasta. The garlic spread is delicious on baked potatoes too, so remember that for later when you are off detox...

To avoid bad garlic breath, just brush and floss carefully after your meal. Rinse with peppermint water. Chew fresh parsley, and your breath smells sweet again.

Enjoy one piece of fresh fruit

Choose between one peach, three apricots or two plums. Cut the fruit into thin slivers; this makes them last longer and taste delicious. Drink one big glass of water with lemon peel (prepare a jug in the morning). Add one teaspoon of ascorbic acid (pure Vitamin C) and one teaspoon of honey.

Evening workout

If you did not follow a complete workout program in the morning, you can do it in the early evening before dinner. You have several programs to choose from, so try them and find out which one is best for you. Find music that gives you energy and makes you want to move.

Remember that it's the moving, stretching and lifting that will shape your body, increase your metabolism, and rejuvenate your body and your total looks.

Detox dinner choices

You can enjoy steamed cauliflower, broccoli, parsnips, kale, carrots, asparagus or leeks, with lots of chopped parsley and/ or any kind of onions baked in the oven or lightly blanched in olive oil. Combine the vegetables you prefer and add new kinds gradually. Add herbs and spices if you like for extra taste and nutrition.

Steamed vegetables can also be mixed into filling soups. Just keep the mineral rich water from steaming and thicken it with some corn flour mixed with cold water. You can also make any kind of mixed salad for dinner during the detox period if you prefer cold food.

Vitamins and mineral supplements

After dinner, take a complete vitamin-mineral supplement, and also an extra B-complex tablet. I also recommend 400 IU of Vitamin E to rejuvenate your skin and improve your general health and energy. To increase a sluggish metabolism, it's very smart to add a kelp supplement.

Evening Ritual

Cleanse your skin until it sparkles and pamper it with oil and cream. Clean your teeth, gums and tongue religiously. It's extremely important to brush properly every morning and evening and always floss and/or use mini brushes to get rid of all the plaque. Remember to scrape your tongue too as a lot of germs can hide in all the tiny crevices.

Lots of teeth are lost to gum diseases that are hard to detect until it's too late. Hidden infections can ruin your jawbone too, so get hold of the best dentist you can afford to prevent problems (or cure the existing ones).

Regular check-ups and treatments are a must and a priority even if they are expensive. They will likely save you money (and your smile…) in the long run.

If you want to disinfect and kill even the most difficult germs, rinse with hydrogen peroxide at least once a day. It's a fabulous antiseptic, even for anaerobic bacteria that lurk in the gums and around the roots. It's also the number one teeth whitener. Ask in the pharmacy for the right dilution.

Oil pulling for total health

To further strengthen and improve the condition of your teeth and gums, it's recommended to use white oil swilling. After cleaning, pour some sesame oil (or coconut or olive oil) into your mouth, and swill it around until it turns white!

This is an ancient Ayurvedic method of killing germs and getting healthy gums and teeth, as well as healing and preventing all kinds of infections in all parts of your body.

Chapter 9

YOU ARE WHAT YOU EAT

Your skin is a reflection of your eating habits

The health and functionality of all your cells depends on what kind of fuel you serve them. Beautiful food will mean that they surface looking plump and will feel like new when they get all they need to function properly in a clean and oxygen-rich environment. Your skin renews itself every three to four weeks.

What you provide your cells with today will show in the mirror in less than a month. Will it be a glowing NEW you or will it be the tired, ageing version because you have postponed the start of your new life? I think you have intelligence and self respect to go for it.

Invest four weeks in your New You, and be rewarded with a natural, amazing makeover.

Lifestyle Diets

After a few detox days, start following one of my lifestyle eating plans. The plans are based on the right choice of foods and beverages and food supplements to ensure you fill your body with all the vitamins and minerals that are crucial to health and beauty. You will not starve or feel deprived. You will be eating a lot of great, nutritious food put together in delicious daily menus. It's not complicated. This food is very easy and fun to make and a pleasure to eat.

You will not count calories or carbohydrates, and you will gradually learn to rely on your own eye for measuring ingredients.

You will also learn to adjust the portions to your own metabolism and level of activity, as you weigh and measure yourself once a week. If you are not satisfied with the weight loss, then you are eating more than you are burning off.

It's your daily eating habits that will shape your body, health, energy level and skin, and determine your looks in general. It's your total lifestyle that will be your fountain of youth.

Fill your larders with foods for youth and beauty

I have made a checklist that you can also use as a template for your shopping list. It contains the basics that should be in your kitchen to make the meals in the New You Eating Plan. It gives you a great variety in tastes, prices, and availability. The different daily menus are easy to make, easy to follow, and versatile. You can switch and alter ingredients and easily adjust the taste with different seasonings.

Joy of cooking

It's very important that you make food that tastes delicious for you. This differs greatly from person to person, as everybody has their own food history inherited from their families and local traditions.

The joy of cooking differs greatly from one person to another too, and the eating plan must of course be adjusted to that. It's so important that you make the plan your own, and that you find out exactly how you can use the ingredients to create your own healthy and tasty dishes.

Flexible eating plans for one or more

You have probably noticed that I am focusing on you as a mature person, not a mother with growing children or teenagers. That is another story, another concept.

This book and my NEW YOU plan is aimed at you, whether you are single, married, or in a relationship. The eating plans can easily be adjusted to two (or more) people and the portions can of course just be increased, and other food added as needed. This way, you can eat meals together.

I know a lot of women with husbands and children who have followed the eating plan this way, and the whole family has ended up healthier, slimmer, and fitter. The husbands lose their potbellies, normalise their blood pressure, cholesterol and blood sugar level without even realising they have been on a healthy eating plan.

Heal yourself with good nutrition

Many people suffering from a wide variety of our most common (and deadly) illnesses would probably be far better o on the right foods and making small adjustments to their everyday lifestyle than popping pills. How long does suppressing the signals of the body last, and at what cost?

In the Western world, many don't realise they are sending themselves to an early grave. How bad is our ignorance of how our bodies work and what they need! We take less care of our most valuable asset than we do of our cars. Who on earth would fill a petrol car with diesel?

Use my different healthy lifestyle eating plans and menus for permanent weight loss until you know exactly what you can and should eat. Use them to help you choose ingredients and meals for you and your family.

The idea of this book is to inspire and teach you how to cook healthier without losing the pleasure of good foods and delicious eating. I advise you to write down your own menus and recipes as you follow mine.

You can add and subtract and make them your own specialities with different herbs and spices.

Remember: A lot of traditional dishes can be much healthier when we reduce fat and sugar and use less of starchy carbohydrates like potatoes, corn, beans, lentils, pasta and rice. Modernize them and make them even tastier as you carry your food culture into the modern world.

Chapter 10

THE NEW YOU QUICK WEIGHT LOSS DIET

This is a great eating plan to start with, and I recommend it for the first week on your New You plan. It's diuretic and cleansing for the body, and it's really easy to follow. This plan is also great for regular detox if you feel bloated or just feel the need to eat light.

Morning

Before breakfast

- *1 big glass of diluted lime juice or lemon juice*

- *1 teaspoon of olive oil*

Breakfast

- *1 hardboiled egg*

- *1 full grain crisp bread*

- *1 grated carrot with freshly pressed orange juice*

- *1/2 grapefruit (can be grilled if you like hot food)*

- *Coffee or tea (with hot milk if you prefer it). If you like it sweet, add Stevia according to your taste.*

Midmorning

- *1 big cup of peppermint tea with a drop of honey*

- *1/2 apple cut into thin slices*

Lunch every day

- *Green salad, any kind, as much as you like*

- *1 hardboiled egg*

- *2 tomatoes*

- *1/2 grapefruit*

- *1 crisp bread with 1/2 banana*

- *Tea or coffee (with milk and Stevia if you prefer it)*

Afternoon

- *1 big slice of melon or 1 orange*

- *1 cup of hibiscus tea (or other kind of fruit tea)*

Dinner casseroles and stews

You have three main choices. The first one is vegetarian, the second is based on fish and seafood, and the third is based on chicken. Because of all the ingredients in a stew, it contains all the valuable nutrients that usually just going down the drain when you strain vegetables. This way your body will get filled to the brim with minerals, vitamins, and valuable roughage that cleanse and restore your body.

You can gradually be more creative in the kitchen and make lots of your own specialties with different variations in taste and texture. But to start with my best advice is to keep it simple and get used to this lean and healthy way of cooking.

The base for all the casseroles is pure vegetable stock (cubes or powder), water, and the ingredients cut into cubes and slices. Add some sea salt, pepper and the spices you prefer. Garlic is super healthy, and great in all the different casseroles. If you prefer a thicker, gravy-like base, you can use corn flour to make it extra yummy.

Green stew

Carrots, celery, kale, onions, leek, potatoes, and any other vegetable you can think of. Add lots of finely chopped parsley before serving.

Fish and Seafood Stew

Onions, potatoes, leek and carrots go nicely with fish and seafood. Dill is great for extra taste.

Chicken (or lean meat) stew

Corn, sweet red peppers, onions, leek, cauliflower, peas and green beans are tasty. Add some basil or other green herbs if you like.

You can add more water to all the stews and turn them into delicious soups. This is great for filling your stomach, prolonging the meal, and offers more variation. If you like, you can also have a green salad as a starter.

Eat in style

It's very important to enjoy your meals, and the way you serve them is part of a way of living. Eating should be a pleasure for the eyes as well as your taste buds and offer much more than just filling you up. Pamper yourself by arranging nice table setting for your meals and make the most out of enjoying your food.

Use candles and flowers, nice tablemats or tablecloths, your beautiful glasses and cutlery, and arrange the food on your plate just like a chef would do it.

While the stew is simmering, change for dinner. Go into the bathroom, have a good look in the mirror, and spend five minutes to refresh your look. Brush and style your hair, put on some makeup, spray on a touch of your most expensive perfume and change into a nice outfit that feels comfortable (including shoes).

Put on some soft music to put you in a good mood and relax and enjoy your meal without hurrying. Take time to savour the different tastes and flavours.

You should eat in style – even if you live alone.

Lots of us have beautiful china, silver and glassware that we only use on special occasions. Lots of us only bother to dress and put on makeup when we have company.

This is actually quite a bleak and depressing way of living, but it's an important aspect of self-respect to get out of the passivity and make an effort for your New You.

Make every day a special day in your new life. Do the little extras to make you look good and feel good and give yourself the assurance that you are worth it.

Healthy drinks and cocktails

When you are on detox or trying to lose weight, wine and drinks with alcohol are a no-no. Give your liver a chance to cleanse itself and rebuild tissues.

Be aware that lots of medicines are hard on the liver too, so even if you are a non-drinker, your liver needs a detox and a rest to rejuvenate and repair itself. Here are some healthy drink alternatives that will help to flush out even more toxins and also rehydrate your body.

Fizzy long drinks and fruity cocktails

Mix any kind of fresh fruit juice with fizzy mineral water. Use beautiful glasses and add ice cubes or crushed ice. The ultimate is of course to have a juicer and make the natural drinks from scratch. All kinds of citrus fruits are particularly nice in fizzy drinks. Decorate – if possible - with fresh mint; it's tasty and very aromatic.

Iced Tea

Hibiscus, red berries, apple and cinnamon, caramello and vanilla, peppermint: the choices are endless, so you just have to hunt for your special favourites. Make strong tea, keep it in the fridge, and serve it in long glasses with ice cubes and a twist of lemon, a strawberry and a slice of cucumber or cherries.

Iced Coffee

If you are a coffee person, you will probably enjoy coffee with ice cubes in a long glass with or without milk. It's a great alternative if you are out in the evening, as it's free of calories and alcohol.

Spa Water

Water with slices of fruit is delicious. In luxurious spas all over the world you find carafes with this healthy, tasty water. It's so easy to copy at home! Here are some of my favourites: Lemon (or lime) water with slices of fresh lemon, cucumber water, orange water, pineapple water and strawberry water.

I also use fresh herbs in water; it's very tasty and healthy. Try fresh mint leaves, sprigs of rosemary and thyme, or basil, just to mention a few. Just use your imagination.

Learn to eat like a slim person

This is not a diet; it's an eating plan, a lifestyle plan, where food is nutrition, energy and the provider of all the essential nutrients that you need to live your life in the best possible way. To make it simple, I have put this plan together with different choices for breakfast and lunch, and the dinners are based on the healthy ingredients that I recommend on a regular basis.

This eating plan will teach you to choose and combine what is good for you and exclude the fattening, unhealthy elements of your daily diet. If you follow it closely, it's easy to adjust it to what you like, what you are used to, and actually tailor make your own menu gradually.

Chapter 11

NEW YOU FAMILY DIET

As you will notice, nothing in my menus is based on exact measurements or weighing, nor on counting calories or carbohydrates. It's not my philosophy, and I think it's the wrong approach to life to limit it with details.

It's much more important that you learn to adjust your food and drink intake to what your body needs, to your individual metabolism whether it's high or low - and to automatically choose the right ingredients for healthy eating and cooking.

I hope the eating plan will gradually become an ingrained part of your life, so you can automatically choose what is good for you and steer clear of the non-nutritious foods. After The Detox and the Quick Loss Diet, I recommend that you stay on the New You Easy Diet for a week or two.

Learn to cook for slimming down and health

Be very conscious of your ingredient choices and how you cook them because it's so important that you learn what works for your new lifestyle. The eating plans are only to help and inspire until you learn how to plan your meals and the way you cook, so that you – at the end of the four week New You transformation program, will be so happy with the result that your new lifestyle will be part of your life forever.

Hopefully, you will also be a source of inspiration for your friends and family, and a living example of the benefits of nutrition, exercise, and personal care as the best way of getting younger, healthier, and really beautiful no matter what age you are.

Easy Diet breakfast choices

Choose the kind of breakfast you prefer. You know your body, so you know what is best for your metabolic type. Do not accept that everybody has to eat a big breakfast to be healthy and happy. We are different, and a lot of new research and health professionals confirm that breakfast is not a key to getting slim and healthy. So, listen to your body - it often knows best.

If you dislike breakfast, fine. Choose the light version just to get your metabolism going after sleeping. You can also vary between the four choices during the week. It's up to you what makes you feel happy while still losing the weight and inches you want.

Supplements are a must

Vitamin and mineral supplement, after you have finished eating, are a must in my opinion. You also need a daily dose of unsaturated fat. You can choose between different oils. As an oil supplement, I am a serious fan of cold pressed olive oil (choose the best quality you can a afford), and I use it as a supplement and a skincare oil, as well as in cooking.

Fish oils (Omega 3) are also very beneficial for your health. As a Norwegian, I know that cod liver oil has always been the number one supplement. It tastes horrid, and as a child I could never get it down without rushing to the bathroom. Even touching a bottle in the fridge made me throw up.

Today there are many different fish oils in capsules and though they are good for you, it's also important to eat fat fish a couple of times a week in addition to using supplements.

Basic everyday breakfast

- *2 multigrain crisp breads with as much roughage as possible*

- *Tea or coffee without sugar or cream*

- *Health juice: 1 medium glass orange juice/water with 1 teaspoon ascorbic acid (pure Vitamin C).*

- *Choose between the four following extras on your crisp bread*

1. For those who dislike breakfast

- *2 big spoons of cottage cheese. Slices of a tomato and cucumber*

- *1 small glass of skimmed milk*

2. For those who like cereals and milk

- *1 small low-fat unsweetened yoghurt*

- *1 handful of oats*

- *Some fresh fruit or berries*

3. For those who are hungry in the morning

- *2 eggs served scrambled or as omelette, poached, hard or soft boiled*

- *1 slice of chicken or other lean meat*

- *1 small glass of skimmed milk*

4. For those who like a hot breakfast

- *1 hard- or soft-boiled egg*

- *1 slice of low fat, yellow, hard cheese*

- *Slices of tomato and cucumber*

- *1 small glass of skimmed milk*

If you choose the big breakfast number 3, you must restrict your intake (smaller portions) for lunches and dinners.

Use common sense and follow your weight. If it stays at the same level but you want to reduce it, you have to cut down your intake or use much more energy for physical exercise.

Choose your lunch

If you work, you will have to prepare your lunch and bring it with you. The best thing is to do it before you go to bed, put it in the fridge, and grab it in the morning before you leave. If you are working at home, retired, or a homemaker, you can make lots of low-calorie delicious lunches. For drinks, it's tea or coffee, ice water or lemon water (add some sweetener if you must but try Stevia for a healthy sugar substitute).

1. Brown bag

- *1 slice brown full grain bread (as much roughage as possible)*

- *1 slice low fat yellow cheese*

- *1 tomato*

- *Cucumber, as much as you like*

- *1 orange*

This is easy to make as a sandwich. You can also cut your tomato and cucumber, mix it with leaves of green salad, and keep it fresh in a plastic container. Eat the orange in parts, including the white pith inside the skin as it's brimming with vital bioflavonoids.

2. Salads

You can use any kind of leafy green salad or finely sliced cabbage. Add cut tomatoes, cucumber, sweet peppers and chopped onions (or any other vegetables you like).

Dressing

Mix a little olive oil, apple cider vinegar or lemon juice with herbs, salt and pepper. Add some milk, garlic and mustard if you like a spicy dressing. Keep the salad in a plastic container and the dressing in a separate bottle so you can add it before eating to avoid a soggy salad. For variation during the week you can add tuna fish, chicken, lean ham or eggs.

Afternoon snack

One peeled carrot and one stalk of leek can be a crunchy extra afternoon snack. Drink lots and lots of water during the day, and bring a big bottle of your favourite herbal tea to sip on. It all helps to keep you hydrated, satisfied, and full of energy.

Lunch at home

1. Grilled Cheese Sandwich

Make a delicious hot grilled cheese and tomato sandwich and serve it with a nice orange and cucumber salad as a side dish. Add some chopped onion for extra taste.

2. French Omelette

Make a French omelette with 2 eggs mixed with 2 spoons of water and a touch of salt. Pour into a hot Teflon frying pan, lift the edges of the egg mixture and tilt the pan so the uncooked egg floats under until all is set and deliciously light golden brown. You can fill it with finely sliced red sweet peppers or sliced mushrooms and chopped onions. Chopped leak and/or chopped chicken or lean meat leftovers are also great for fillings. Fry the filling in a separate frying pan or fry them first and then add the eggs.

Use your imagination and listen to your taste buds. Green salad is nice as a side dish. As a dessert you can enjoy a fruit salad with half an apple mixed with half a grapefruit cut up into small pieces.

3. Seafood or chicken salad

All kinds of fish and seafood are super healthy and make great additions to salads. Tuna and salmon are probably the easiest choices and taste wonderful with different kinds of leafy greens, onions, a little garlic, tomatoes, and whatever other vegetables you like.

I prefer a white, creamy dressing made of yoghurt, mixed with a little sugar or Stevia to soften it, and with lots of garlic, finely chopped onions, a touch of mustard, salt and pepper. You can use chicken as a substitute for seafood.

4. Stir fry

Make a salad with leafy greens and use the rest in a stir fry. The same ingredients in a hot pan with a little oil makes them crunchy, delicious, and an excellent accompaniment to green salad.

5. Soups and stews

This is my first choice of nutritious, low-calorie, tasty and filling dinners. You can vary these endlessly according to your preferences and taste buds. The stews are perfect for anyone who likes to feel really full, satisfied, and not the victim of a severely restricted diet with mini portions.

Like my mother said: I am tired of Air Soup and Waiting Burgers (she was always on a diet due to a metabolic disorder combined with a healthy appetite).

She finally lost lots and lots of weight – and gained lots of healthy years by following my system – and eating her fill of vegetable stews. The more she chewed – the more she lost....

Basic New You stew

Choose hard vegetables like carrots, turnip, pumpkin, celery roots: The more variation, the better. Add onions, leeks, garlic, parsley, and go wild in the green department. Chop everything into nice squares.

Fill up a big pot with enough salted water to cover the ingredients. Simmer gently and add more salt and herbs according to your taste. You can also use stock cubes to add taste.

If you make the soups or stews from the right ingredients, you can eat absolutely as much as you can get into your body. If you like the stew thicker and "creamier", you mix corn flour with cold water and add it until you reach the consistency you want. The New You Diet will actually give you a three-course dinner. How about that for slimming!

Three course New You dinner

Starters for one week

1. Raw food grated vegetables with lemon with a little honey

2. Green, mixed salad. Vinaigrette dressing with or without garlic

2. Broth with chopped parsley and/or finely chopped white onion

3. Broth with finely sliced mushrooms, onions and garlic

4. 1/2 a grapefruit, grilled

5. 3 thin slices of honey melon with grated ginger

6. Asparagus (white or green) with sea salt

7. 1 big grilled tomato (2 halves) with pepper, salt, garlic, parsley

Main course

Choose one portion of meat, fowl or fish. The size should be similar to a deck of cards. If it's lean fish, you can have a slightly larger portion. Remove visible fat on meat. How you prepare it is up to you, as your eating habits, cooking traditions and cultural background will give you a set of preferences.

Salad, steamed or grilled vegetables on the side

Choose whatever you like from the vast choice of vegetables in your supermarket. You can eat them in ample portions, and combine them with the fish, meat or fowl. You can steam, wok or boil the vegetables, but keep them at dense and do not make mash of them.

Drink lots of water, with ice if you like. Add slices of lemon, orange, cucumber or berries if you want more taste.

Dessert

Enjoy one fresh fruit. Vary your choice to give new experiences. You can also bake and grill fruit and make them even tastier with a touch of cinnamon.

Remember to eat in style

Dress the table and arrange the food professionally because you deserve it! Put on cool background music and relax with a nice frozen fruit or berry cocktail before you eat. Use your time, enjoy and savour it, and feel that you really deserve the best.

Eat like a slim person, eat like a celebrity...

That means slowly, chewing every bite, enjoying the different tastes and textures in the slimming, healthy meal. It's really all about being a slim and healthy gourmet; not a fat, greedy gourmand.

Chapter 12

NEW YOU CLASSIC DIET

This is my favourite eating plan as it follows the basic guidelines for a healthier way of eating. I have used the principles for creating lots and lots of dishes and menus.

This way of eating is suitable for anyone who wants to eat healthier, get slimmer and learn really good eating habits, which means they won't put on the lost kilograms again. Why? Because this plan can be customised to anyone, anywhere! It's adaptable and versatile whether you are single or have a family and children, whether you are a busy businesswoman or a full-time mum.

Adapt the diet to your style of life

This flexible diet can be varied indefinitely, but you may want to follow it to the letter, particularly in the beginning. Once you become familiar with the ingredients and way of cooking, it's very easy for you to make your own weekly menus.

Creativity, common sense and know-how are the spices you need to make healthy foods with less fat, sugar, additives and empty calories for you and your family, because healthy foods are the best preventive medicine.

Let me stress that this is a healthy diet that everyone benefits from-whether they need to lose weight or not. Those who do not need to lose weight can add extra servings of the main dish and add potatoes, rice, pasta, sauces, etc. They should just adjust the size of servings according to their needs.

However, if one person is overweight in a family, it tends to be a problem for several members, as it's a reflection of the family's lifestyle. It's also a difficult subject to discuss, as most overweight people are very sensitive about the subject, so even if you have decided to get healthier and slimmer together, be careful what you say.

Healthy eating sounds better than diet

Sometimes it's better NOT to tell others you are on a diet. You can just tell them that you feel tired, sluggish, and you need to make healthier food choices and consume more nutrients for more energy. You can always tell a white lie if you want to encourage others to join you. Tell them that you have painful problems with your stomach, intestines etc., and you have to eat more sensibly, and undertake regular detox. You don't have to tell them it's a diet; just that you will make healthier food.

Bye, bye belly

Countless women following this plan have been impressed with how delicious the food is. Many of their husbands have eliminated their dangerous potbelly without feeling they've missed anything. Women have explained that their husbands felt slimmer, healthier and more energetic week by week, that they loved the food, and did not realise they had been on a diet.

Good advice

Always serve water, preferably with ice and lemon slice, with all meals. Drink a glass of water with thin slices of apple or lemon before breakfast too as this can stimulate the immune system and fat burning. Drink as much tea and coffee as you like. If you like milk in coffee and tea, choose the low-fat version. Also, chew on raw vegetables between meals.

Choose between seven breakfasts

1. For those who like cheese

- *1 slice of full grain bread, 1 slice of low-fat yellow cheese or 3 tablespoons Cottage cheese*

- *1 crisp bread, slices of tomatoes and cucumber*

- *1 small glass of low-fat milk (preferably kefir)*

2. For those with a sweet tooth

- *1 slice of full grain bread with 1/2 a small banana mashed as spread*

- *1 egg, 1 glass of low-fat milk*

3. For those who like cereals

- *1/2 cup oats or unsweetened cereal*

- *1 glass of light milk or 1 small cup of Greek, unsweetened yoghurt*

- *1 apple or 1 orange*

4. For those who like smoothies

- *1 egg, 1/2 glass of low-fat milk, 3 tablespoons of berries, apples, pears or carrots, 1 large spoon of oats. Blend the ingredients until smooth and creamy.*

5. For those who like sandwiches

- *2 slices of bread with egg and tomato, 1 grapefruit or orange, 1 glass of milk*

6. For those who like fruit:

- *Fruit salad of 1/2 apple, 1/2 orange, 1/2 grapefruit or other types of fresh fruit or berries. 2 tablespoons of yogurt sprinkled with cereal.*

7. For those who love eggs

- *1 crisp bread.*

Choose a new lunch pack every day

It can be a challenge to eat a healthy, slim lunch when you are working. Do it the Norwegian way and make lunch at home and bring it to the office. It saves you a lot of money compared to going out to restaurants for your lunch, and you have total control over what you eat.

If you want to get out of the office for your lunch break, have your lunch at your desk first or bring it with you to the nearest park. Use the lunch break to go for brisk walks and get into shape too. It's great for your body and brain.

Easy does it

I have different alternatives that are healthy, filling, fast and simple. They will keep you satisfied until you get home, and it will prevent low blood sugar and cravings.

Norwegian Brown Bag lunches

The principle is to make sandwiches with 2 thin slices of full grain bread with different kinds of fillings. Add some salad, vegetables and a little fruit for healthy, low calorie lunches.

1. Mackerel is healthy all year round

- *2 slices of bread with mackerel in tomato and slices of cucumber. This saltwater fish provides you with very important nutrients, like fatty Omega 3 acids and first class proteins. If you don´t like mackerel, I recommend tuna. It's tasty and also very healthy. Most people don´t eat enough fish, so please try this for lunch as often as possible.*

2. Eggs and cheese give you protein

- *1 slice of brown bread with egg and tomato slices. 1 crisp bread with low fat cheese and slices of sweet, red bell peppers.*

3. Sandwich salad filling

- *2 slices of full grain bread with homemade filling of thin slices of cabbage, raw grated carrots mixed with a little low-fat mayo and yoghurt. Add low fat ham if you like.*

4. Tasty chicken sandwich

- *1 slice of coarse bread with slices of chicken breast, cucumber and tomatoes.*

- *1 crisp bread with cottage cheese and thin slices of apple.*

5. Simple and fast

- *1 cup of yoghurt natural with cereal and 1 apple.*

6. Cheese and ham

- *1 slice of brown bread with lettuce, a slice of lean ham, cucumber and tomatoes.*

- *1 crisp bread with lean yellow cheese (or cottage cheese) and slices of red bell peppers.*

7. Grilled ham and cheese sandwich

- *2 slices of brown bread filled with low fat yellow cheese, a thin slice of ham, and a little mustard. Grill it, cut into four sections, and serve with a little salad and an orange for dessert. Hot food feels more filling, so remember that most sandwiches can be grilled. These are great for the days you are at home.*

Vegetable snacks

If you know your willpower is weak and your cravings are too strong to resist, it's very important that you can put something in your mouth and chew every time the urge hits you.

The best way is actually very simple: Cut up a lot of vegetables at home and bring them to work in a plastic bag. Every time you feel you MUST have something, grab the bag and chew, chew, chew. Sticks of carrots, celery, turnip (and all kinds of hard root vegetables) are excellent.

Another good tip is to keep a packet of healthy crisp bread in your office drawer. Break off a piece when you need to chew something. You are not really hungry; it's far more a mental than physical hunger.

Fill up your stomach with plenty of water during the day. It revitalises you, rehydrates all your cells, and it's excellent for a youthful looking skin. It's also extremely important for improved circulation and detoxifying your body.

Choose from 7 salads for lunch

Whether you are at home or at work, salads are delicious for lunch. Remember, you can treat yourself to quite large portions if you are very careful with the dressings you use. Get a lunch box that holds exactly one portion size. Grab a small bottle for your low-cal dressing as well.

You can have crispbread with sesame seeds on the side. These taste great and give you lots of useful dietary fibre with few calories. Personally, I think these are a great alternative to ordinary bread to maintain good digestion and normal weight.

Dressing no 1 for these salads: Yoghurt (or kefir) sweetened with Stevia and spiced up with a touch of salt and mustard. You can cut up fresh herbs and add more taste to the dressing if you like.

Dressing no 2: A little olive oil mixed with lemon juice or vinegar, salt and pepper, herbs according to taste – a touch of Stevia, and a little low-fat milk.

1. Cabbage coleslaw style

Slice cabbage into very thin slices (use a mandolin if you have one). Add finely cut onions. Grate carrots, celery and any other greens you like. Be creative and make your own specialties.

2. Chicken salad

Cut chicken into fine pieces. Approximately 1/2 a cup is suitable for a salad portion. Mix with cubes of celery. Tear up plain lettuce leaves or use finely chopped iceberg salad. Cut up 1/4 of an apple and add 4 walnuts for extra taste.

3. Tuna salad

Cut iceberg lettuce in strips, finely cut onions, add olives, cubed cucumber and a small tin of tuna in oil or water. Mix well. Decorate with a hardboiled egg divided in half after dressing. Lemon adds extra taste.

4. Tomato and mozzarella salad

2 large tomatoes cut into thin slices and add salt and pepper. I also recommend a little garlic powder for extra flavour. Spread the tomatoes on a big plate and add thinly sliced onion rings and wafer-thin slices of mozzarella. Add some fresh basil and a touch of olive oil. Serve a slice of full grain bread on the side.

5. Spinach salad

It's easy to forget about the super-healthy spinach, as many think it's not suitable for salads, but it has a really good taste. It's delicious with strips of smoked salmon and boiled egg, but you can mix it with almost all kinds of leftovers of meat and sh. Spinach goes very well with hard fruit like apples and pears too.

6. Mixed vegetables and fruit salad

All raw vegetables and fruits have lots of fibre, vitamins and minerals, as well as great taste. All of the natural nutrients are preserved in a natural balance when eaten raw too. Just pick from the vegetable and fruit dish (choose organic as much as possible). You can mix everything and vary the dressings. Curry powder, cilantro, rosemary and thyme add interesting tastes.

Avoid the perfect fruits!

Shy away from the perfect, shiny apples and other fruits that look identical and artificial. These glossy fruits are covered with silicone and have to be soaked in water with vinegar before you can eat them. My best advice is don't buy them!! Choose fruit and vegetables that are natural and less perfect. Organic is perhaps a little bit more expensive, but so much better for you!

7. Cucumber salad

This sweet and sour cucumber salad is a winner, and delicious as a side dish when you serve steamed or grilled fish. I also think it's a delicious accompaniment for spicy food in general, and I usually make large portions to store in a glass jar in the fridge. It contains minimal calories as I sweeten it with Stevia.

Mix water and white vinegar to the strength you like. Add some salt and sweeten it with Stevia to taste. Don't be afraid to experiment. Should you get the wrong mix, just pour it out and start over again until you get it right. The ingredients cost almost nothing.

Wash a cucumber and cut it into very thin slices with a knife or a mandolin. Cover the slices completely with the dressing and store it for a couple of hours in the fridge.

Delicious basic dinners

1. Pork with mushrooms

Season a small pork fillet with salt, pepper and garlic. Put some butter in a frying pan (or grill pan), wait until it browns then fry the fillet quickly. Add sliced mushrooms. Serve with a small baked potato and a large serving of green salad.

2. Steamed fish fillet

Salt the fish and let it steam in a little boiled water with added lemon. Serve with two small boiled potatoes and one boiled carrot, cucumber salad and a large portion of green lettuce salad with yoghurt or kefir dressing.

3. Vegetable casserole

Cut up different vegetables such as celery, carrots, turnip, leeks and onions. Make a vegetable broth in a saucepan then add the vegetables and let them boil until soft (but firm to chew). Cut some parsley or other green herbs and add. Thicken the stew with corn flour in cold water. Serve with crisp bread.

4. Baked vegetables

Put 1 cup of boiled, long grain rice and as much frozen (thawed) vegetable mix as you like in an ovenproof dish. Whisk 2 or 3 eggs with 2 to 3 tablespoons of water, salt, pepper and spices and pour the mixture over the rice and vegetables. Place in the oven at 200 degrees until it's golden. Serve with a slice of full grain bread with lean ham.

5. Vegetarian pizza

Cover readymade plain pizza dough with lots of sliced tomatoes, squash, finely chopped onion or leek, and slices of mushroom. Season with salt, pepper, and some fresh herbs and garlic. Add a little grated low-calorie yellow cheese as a topping. Place in the oven at 200 degrees and serve with a plain green salad with a simple oil and vinegar dressing. Have one fruit of your choice cut into slices for dessert.

6. Baked chicken fillet with asparagus

Cut 1 chicken fillet open and season well with garlic, pepper and salt. Fill it with asparagus (fresh or canned) and put it in an ovenproof dish together with thin sliced potato. Bake until crisp and golden and serve with as much mixed salad as you can eat with a light dressing.

7. Filled fish in foil

You can fill any kind of fish with lots of finely chopped onions and other vegetables. Don't forget to salt it well. You can vary the dish by filling with prawns, asparagus, and/or mushrooms. This is delicious with a small portion of boiled potatoes and steamed vegetables, such as carrots, broccoli or asparagus as side dishes.

Serve with a white low-fat sauce with finely chopped chives. Sweet and sour cucumber salad is also tasty as a side dish.

Be a creative cook

These are just a few examples of healthy and lean dishes that give you lots of useful nutrients. They are easy to prepare and all the ingredients are available anywhere at an affordable prices.

Eat slowly, eat less

It's smart to start your meal with a crispy green salad, some raw food, oven-grilled vegetables or a vegetable broth with fresh herbs. This gives your brain enough time to register that your stomach is full. It takes about 20 minutes.

New You Slim Dressings

Dressings often add a lot of extra calories to a meal. It's important that you are aware of that and make your own low-calorie dressing. My recipes are simple, tasty, low fat, and sugar free. Many commercial dressings have lots of fat, sugar, salt, and additives. You get a far better taste if you make your own.

French dressing

Use a glass jar with a tight lid to make the basic dressing that can be varied indefinitely. You can make a large portion, because it keeps well in the fridge.

The classic recipe has 2/3 oil and 1/3 wine or lemon juice. To reduce fat and calories, I mix with water: 1/3 of good quality cold-pressed olive oil, 1/3 white wine vinegar and 1/3 of water. Add salt, pepper, garlic, 1 teaspoon of mustard and extra herbs. Give it some sweetness with a touch of Stevia. Experiment until you find your favourite blend.

Mediterranean herbal dressing

Use the basic oil-vinegar-water dressing from the previous recipe and add salt, pepper, garlic, and finely chopped fresh basil, parsley, and dried oregano.

Curry Dressing

Add 2 teaspoons of curry powder and 2 teaspoons of finely chopped onions. You can add a little mango chutney for a more exotic, fuller taste.

Italian dressing

Add 1 clove of freshly pressed garlic to a finely chopped onion and add 1 tablespoon of finely chopped red bell pepper. You can add chopped basil if you like variation.

Chili dressing

Mix sweet chili sauce with the basic dressing above. You can make it hotter by adding red peppers.

Classic white dressing

Replace the water in the basic recipe with low fat milk and add mustard, garlic, and Stevia for sweetness. This has been a favourite in our family for years and many people have requested our "secret" recipe. Now you have it. Enjoy!

Yoghurt dressing

Use Greek yogurt mixed with low fat milk to the right texture. Sweeten it with a little Stevia. The more fluid it is, the fewer calories you get, as very little is needed to cover vegetables. You can vary this in many ways.

Fish and shellfish dressing

Use the basic yoghurt dressing and add a little tomato ketchup, garlic, finely chopped onions, and dill.

Oslo dressing

Add lots of finely chopped chives to the basic yoghurt-milk dressing. This is a delicious dressing, particularly for lettuce, salads with fish, fowl and meat dishes.

Roquefort dressing

Crumble a little Roquefort cheese into the yogurt dressing and whisk until creamy. You can use s blender to get an extra smooth dressing.

Creative cuisine

Fish and seafood are very healthy and excellent when you want to lose weight. They are an excellent source of protein and fatty fish contain very important fatty acids that are beneficial for your heart and circulatory system. Here are some straightforward recipes for a healthy diet.

Filled fish in foil

This is one of my favourites as it's amazingly simple and easy whether in small portions or for company. You can use fish fillets or whole fish that have been cleaned. Lay the fish on a sheet of foil, salt it lightly and add a finely chopped mixture of different ingredients. If using a whole fish, add the filling into the abdomen. Bring the foil together so that it holds the shape and bake at 220 degrees in the oven for 10- 15 minutes for fillets.

Here are suggestions for different fillings:

- Finely chopped onions or leeks

- Asparagus and spring onions

- Mushrooms and finely chopped onions

- Shrimp, lemon slices, and dill

- Chives

You can also make a more Spanish type filling, with tomatoes, paprika, onions, garlic and finely chopped olives. Just use your imagination!

Side dishes

Boiled potatoes, steamed vegetables, carrots (cooked or grated as raw food).

Cucumber salad is fresh and delicious with fish as is lettuce with dressing of kefir milk sweetened with a little Stevia.

Gourmet salmon

Place the salmon fillet on foil and cover with a thin layer of sweet, grainy mustard. Sprinkle chopped almonds on top. Fold the foil and bake in the oven for approximately 15- 20 minutes at 220 degrees. Serve with asparagus (preferably fresh white) and a small portion of rice.

Mediterranean fish soup

This is a thick, creamy and rich fish soup because I use corn flour mixed with cold water to thicken it. You can choose your own ingredients and make it your specialty.

Fill a saucepan with water (or fish/sea food broth). Add salt and cubes of carrots, potatoes, onion slices and leek and steam until tender. Add whatever fish, shrimps, and shellfish you like. Let it all simmer until the fish is cooked. Add lots of finely chopped parsley before serving.

Another alternative is an exciting fish soup Italian style with added chopped tomatoes, carrots, potatoes, chopped garlic, and yellow onions.

Indian fish casserole

You can a make a hot, spicy Indian-inspired pot by replacing the potatoes with round grain rice and plenty of curry sauce.

Steamed fish

This is the simplest and fastest fish dinner. Choose your favourite fish, season it with salt and white pepper (if you like). Let it steam in a little boiling, salted water with some lemon juice, dill, chives, or crushed garlic. The choice is yours. Serve it with boiled carrots and a freshly sliced cucumber salad or a green salad with yoghurt dressing with one small boiled potato.

Flounder with capers

Steam a slightly salted cutlet of flounder in a little white wine or water. Thicken the liquid with corn flour to make a creamy sauce. Delicious with white or green asparagus and mashed potatoes (pommes dauphine).

Tuna Surprise

Tuna is a good and cheap alternative to fresh fish. I always have some cans in the house. It's also smart to have cans of mushrooms, as they can be used in a multitude of ways. Here is a dish that you make in a flash: Tuna with mushroom sauce and rice!

You steam 1 cup of long grain rice. While the rice is steaming, you make a mushroom gravy. Open the can of mushrooms and pour the contents into a pan. When it boils, thicken it with 1 heaped spoonful of corn flour mixed with cold water. Season with salt, pepper, spices if you like - and add finely chopped onions.

Stir in the onions and 1/2 cup deep-frozen peas in the sauce. Heat up. Spread the steamed rice on a serving dish. Put the tuna fish on top and cover it all with the mushroom sauce. You can decorate with tomatoes or eggs and parsley. A big slice of pineapple is refreshing for dessert.

Shrimps Scandinavia style

You can buy shrimps fresh or frozen. If you buy the deep-frozen ones, I recommend that you separate them (in cold water) and then steam them for a moment in boiling salty water (it should be as salty as the sea). Add fresh dill for a delicious taste. Cool and serve them with a garnish of thick lemon slices, more fresh dill, and hot crusty bread.

I recommend this easy dip for the peeled shrimps: Mix low fat mayonnaise with a little ketchup and milk. Add some grated lemon peel, grated onion, and a little garlic. As a dessert you can try half a pear with a blue cheese mixed with cottage cheese.

Hot garlic shrimps

You need shrimps, a little olive oil, and a few garlic cloves cut in thin slices. Heat the oil and fry the garlic and the shrimps (with or without the shell). Serve with long grain rice and lemon wedges. The fatty acids in shrimps are important for your immune systems, brain and skin health as well as many metabolic processes.

Don't be afraid of eating fish

Are you afraid of fish being polluted? Even if you read about mercury and contamination, hormones and antibiotics in farmed fish, we cannot cut such an important food from our diet. I think you should enjoy your fish with a good conscience and have it for dinner a couple of days per week.

You need the fatty acids, the nutrients, the proteins and the very important mineral, iodine, which is vital for normal metabolism and thyroid function. The pollution risk is lower than the risk of low thyroid function, especially if you compare it with all the pollutions, we are victim to in our modern society. To counteract it (and pollutions in general), make regular detox a part of your life.

Chapter 13

CREATIVE COOKING BASICS

Here are some super simple dishes for those days when you feel uninspired and don't feel like cooking. These dishes more or less make themselves. Preparation takes just a few minutes and the rest is done in the oven.

You have plenty of time to change into something comfortable, put on a spot of lip gloss and perfume, some relaxing music and light a few candles. Why not make a weekday a special one? Alone – or with company – who cares?

You deserve to eat well and enjoy it in style. So, give it a try. It's part of your New You lifestyle!!

Enjoy!

Roast chicken leg

Take a quarter of a chicken (without skin), raw or grilled, and season well with garlic, pepper and salt. Place in an ovenproof dish with a small potato, seasoned and cut into thin slices. Bake at 200 degrees until crisp and golden. Serve with a tasty side salad.

Filled chicken breast

Cut a pocket in a chicken breast for filling. Spice it to taste and fill it with whatever you like, such as mushrooms and onions, asparagus, pineapples, apples, lemon and oranges, cottage cheese mixed with blue cheese or simply lots of green herbs and parsley. Place in the oven at 220 degrees for 15 to 20 minutes (depending on the size).

Serve with a baked potato (oven baked for approximately 30 minutes) of boiled, long grained rice with steamed vegetables. Enjoy as much mixed salad as you can eat, with a light dressing of course!

Chicken in béchamel sauce

This is also a good and easy everyday dinner. Make a light white sauce with some butter, our and milk. Season with salt, pepper and tarragon.

Put your favourite deep-frozen vegetable mix in an ovenproof dish, pour 3⁄4 of the sauce over them, and add a layer of onion rings (or leeks). Season the sliced chicken breast and place on top. Add the rest of the sauce and bake for about 20 minutes at 220 degrees.

Chicken in white sweet and sour sauce

Heat up a tin of chickpeas, peas and thin slices of carrots in a light white sauce flavoured with dill. You can also make the sauce sour by adding a little vinegar and water sweetened with Stevia. Serve with a small portion of boiled rice, preferably brown.

Delicious chicken salad

Pluck the meat from half a grilled chicken. Discard the skin away as it contains too much fat. Cut the meat into cubes and mix with finely chopped onions, iceberg lettuce, cubes of pineapple, apples, celery and cucumber.

Mix in some yogurt with some pineapple juice and pour it over for a fresh and fruity dressing. Garnish with some walnuts. Enjoy melon for dessert, or make a nice smoothie with melon, yogurt and ice cubes.

Roast pork chops or liver with onion

Spice chops (remove visible fat) with garlic, salt and black pepper. Hammer them with a rolling pin so they become thin and at and will fry and crisp up in seconds.

Cut fine slices of fresh garlic and cubes of apples and fry them together with finely chopped onions in a little brown butter. Fry the meat (or liver). Serve with a large portion of raw grated carrots and salad.

Cold meat and egg salad

Add a tomato, melon cubes, finely chopped onions and hard-boiled eggs to a mix of salad leaves. Dress with a little virgin oil mixed with apple vinegar or lemon juice, salt, pepper and any herbs you like.

Weekend beef, pork or lamb

Friday is the start of the weekend. Why not go for a spicy, tender, delicious beef, lamb chops or a pork fillet? Season well with black pepper, garlic and some salt. The meat can be grilled or fried on high temperature in a little browned butter.

Serve with a baked potato, baked onion, grilled tomatoes and a delicious crispy green salad with French dressing. If you're not a fan of red meat, a chicken fillet is another option. Enjoy with a glass of red wine and a good fruit salad with some chopped nuts for dessert.

Cold cuts

When you have a little extra time for prepping food, it's smart to roast beef, lamb or pork. Season well and bake in the oven. Let it rest and cool down then cut thin slices to keep as cold cuts for sandwiches. Cut the rest into cubes for stews, a stir fry, curries, Thai and Chinese meals. Thicker slices can be used for quick, protein rich dinners, making this very practical and economic.

Extra for the healthy cook

Egg dishes are easy, super delicious and cover your protein needs. You can easily make an omelette of 2 eggs and 2 tablespoons of water, with a little salt and fill it with mushrooms, lean meat or asparagus. Serve with crisp bread.

How about a French omelette with ham and asparagus? Whip 2 or 3 eggs with 2 to 3 tablespoons of water. Season and pour into a hot Teflon pan. Lift the omelette along the edges so that the batter runs under the top. Let it set and get deliciously yellow. When cooked, add asparagus, ham (or whatever you like) on top, and fold it over.

Make a tasty, fresh tomato salad with finely chopped onions and a light dressing as a side dish. Serve with wholegrain bread and a glass of wine or alcohol-free beer if it's the weekend and you feel like a treat. Sliced kiwi and other exotic fruits made into a fresh fruit salad is a delicious and easy dessert.

Tips for removing fat from food

When you make soups and casseroles with meat - including chicken – reduce the calories by skimming of the fatty surface layer when it cools off and discard as it's no good for you. It's loaded with LDL fatty acids that contribute to high cholesterol and radically increase the risk of cardiovascular disease.

You can also put the cooked meat dish in the freezer for a little while. The fat will set on the top and will be easier to remove. If you don't have enough time or room in your freezer, let the dish cool and put in a handful of ice cubes for a few second and then remove them. The ice cubes will be covered in solidi ed fat and you will have a much leaner dish.

Grow sprouts

Do you remember sprinkling seeds on strips of damp cotton that rapidly sprouted and tasted heavenly on fresh bread with real butter? The seeds are loaded with flavours and nutrients, and certainly recommended as an addition to salads, dressings, omelettes and healthy sandwich fillings.

Wheat, soybeans and a variety of other beans, lentils and seeds can sprout that give you extra proteins, vitamins, and minerals. They also add extra taste and texture to salads, sandwiches, and other dishes. You can get lots of inspiration and advice in health food stores or online.

Do you want hot food?

Keep in mind that you can fry vegetables in a wok to create hot salads. Rice and grains like quinoa or noodles are good accompaniments. Keep in mind that you can also make hot fruit salads. They're delicious and actually more satisfying than when served cold.

If you're craving sauces, you can use Greek yogurt as a base and add extra spices, mashed fruits or berries, olives, beetroots, gherkins or other savouries. Cut up your choice and mix it into Greek yoghurt to make a delicious, spicy cold sauce (like tartare).

Get enough proteins for cell repair and renewal

It's important to have one good hot meal per day, with adequate animal protein in the form of meat, fish, shellfish, fowl or eggs. If you are a vegetarian or vegan, plant proteins must be combined to allow the body to form the vital amino acids for the growth and repair of cells and tissues. Beans and pulses are a typical source. Most of the recipes here can be customized if you want to eat completely green.

It is also an increasing selection on tofu and other vegetarian meat substitutes that you should try out. It takes a while to get used to a different way of cooking and new ways of seasoning to make vegetarian taste more widely accepted, but in our new and greener world – the possibilities for plant based living is increasing by the day. Good for us, for our health, for animals - and for the planet.

Just a few green days a week will make a big difference. I have just one very important piece of advice for you: Learn as much as possible about nutrition. Find reliable sources who knows facts – and avoid sources with fanatics that treat green living as a new religion.

Remember: Truth is not black or white, it has all the colours of the rainbow….

Chapter 14

LOOK YOUR BEST EVERY DAY

Food is for the inside, but we also have to pay attention to the outside. This simple Good Morning Program should be part of your daily routine, and I can promise you that you will look and feel amazing if you take the time and effort to follow it. It's far easier and quicker than you think.

Before you put on makeup, you have to start with a clean canvas.

Feel good

1. Get out of bed, stretch like a cat using all your limbs to get the circulation going after a good night's rest. This is how cats stay so strong, flexible and alert, so take a lesson from them in the movement department.

2. Do some deep breathing to get rid of stale air and fill up with clean, fresh oxygen.

3. Then start your day by drinking lots of water to cleanse, purify, and rehydrate your body from within. A couple of large glasses of water will do the trick.

4. Then it's time for brushing and flossing your teeth. Gargle with salty water. Keep a bottle ready in the bathroom. This is far better than any commercial product for disinfecting and firming up your gums.

5. Splash cold water on your face to wake up, kick the circulation into gear, and close the pores! Put on serum and moisturizer.

6. Take a few quick brush strokes trough your hair and put on your fitness gear.

7. Look good – feel good. Look sporty – feel sporty.

Fitness time

Put on your favourite high-energy music and go. Choose the New You Slim Trim Program, Good morning Sun Yoga or just plain walking, jumping, or skipping. Even

if you have very busy mornings, don't use this as an excuse. You just have to get up a little earlier and do at least 20 minutes of movement to firm up and lose inches.

High achievers and successful people start fitness regimes and jogging before six in the morning. Relax, you don't have to be like that, but do take at least 20 – 30 minutes to move your body every day!

Feel good and take a little time to pamper yourself to get ready for a new day, looking your best!

So, get up a little earlier, get your bum in gear, get physical, and feel that kick of energy. After you have finished your morning fitness program, take a minute or two repeating your relaxing affirmations to motivate yourself.

Here's a reminder of those affirmations:

I am (your name) here and now.

I am healthy, happy, young and beautiful.

I love my body; I love my life.

I am saying goodbye to the past.

I welcome my wonderful future!

Shower and nourish

Strip down, admire your body, and be extremely thankful for being fit and flexible enough to do this. Say, Hello body, you are on your way to being fit and firm, losing inches and looking better each day.

Pamper your body under the shower, and softly scrub off dead skin cells and stimulate the production of strengthening elastin and collagen to renew and restore the elasticity of your skin cells and stimulate a youthful glow.

Focus and enjoy the feeling! Be YOU in the moment, not in the past or the future, but be mindful of your life and that you are living here and now.

Feel yourself tingle with increased circulation and energy. Stay in the feeling and continue with a few more minutes of pampering from toe to top. Show your body that you love it the way it is and you will help it to be its very best. Feel the softness of your skin, your curves, and be happy that you are alive.

Your body deserves the best of care and support, so massage it with plenty of body cream or fragrant body oils from your feet up to your neck to rehydrate your skin.

Pamper your body

If you plan to be out in the sun, always remember that you must be protected with high factor UVA and UVB sun lotion. The sun is your friend and kicks your body into producing a lot of the sunshine vitamin D that is crucial for your calcium absorption, your bones, immune system, and neurotransmitter production. But it can also be your worst enemy if you are not sun wise enough to protect yourself from the forceful rays that damage your skin.

Avoid chemical sunscreens. I absolutely recommend Aloe Vera natural products!

The feel-good feeling

You will feel great when you have finished your health and beauty routine and your quality of life will be boosted. The effort you have made for your body and soul will make your day so much better than the lazy alternative.

Remember the awful feeling when you hardly bother to get out of bed? When you stumble to the kitchen in a haze to get coffee to wake you up?

Remember how it feels to look in the mirror and see an ageing, tired woman (Is that really me?) in a shabby bath robe with bleary eyes, a pale, tired face, hair like a crow's nest and breath like a dragon.

Better to be bright eyed and bushy tailed and look forward to this unique day of your life. This day – to use a cliché – is the first one of the rest of your life, so make the most of it. It will never come again.

Face the day

Always start with cleanser and toner (or wipes) and rinse off with lukewarm water followed by lots of cold water to close your pores and stimulate your skin. Notice the glow and clean look you get. Pat your skin a little and massage a rejuvenating serum and an anti- ageing moisturizer into your damp skin.

Always remember to do the same routine on your neck (and preferably your décolleté. Let it totally absorb before you put on makeup.

Start by covering up any pigmentation spots or broken capillaries with tiny strokes of concealer cream (or pencil). Blend it into your skin. If you need more cover, apply it lightly and blend well. Brush blusher on your cheekbones, and a little bit on your forehead, chin, and earlobes.

A touch on your eyelids is also nice and gives you a younger, lifted look too. Even out everything so there are no harsh borders, it must totally blend with your skin. Look how fresh and glowing your face can become in an instant.

Emphasize your eyes with a liner that brings out the colour of your eyes and defines them. Line close to your upper and lower lashes and soften with your fingertip. A pencil is the easiest tool, as you can get it as soft or as defined as you like. Then put on your mascara. Several thin layers will make your lashes long and look natural.

Waterproof mascara is often practical as it stays on even if you laugh until you cry. If your brows need defining, use tiny feathery strokes to give them shape and colour. Remember, less is more, and it should look soft and totally natural.

Use a good long-lasting lip liner to emphasize the shape of your mouth. Be very meticulous to get an absolutely even result. This will also stop your lipstick from bleeding into the tiny lines most of us get as time goes by. Fill in with lipstick. Let it dry for a moment before you apply gloss. When you look great, you feel great.

Looking good makes your day

Put on something functional that makes you feel and look good for the day ahead, whether it's for work, housework, painting, gardening, shopping, going out to meet friends, or just relaxing at home with a good book or other things you enjoy. If you're not working outside the house, please avoid daytime television and surfing social media.

These are extremely addictive, a pointless waste of time, and a fruitless escape from life and reality. Put away your electronic devices and don't be a puppet jumping to the notifications. Make something exciting happen in your own life instead.

Chapter 15

ALL IN LOVE WITH YOUR LIFE
AND NEW POSSIBILITIES

Back to you, your real life, your health, looks and wellbeing. Since you have bought this book, you obviously take an interest in yourself and your body, and you have a real intention of improving it. A New You means the best and longest lasting version of you.

Enjoy your life

"Live like you will die tomorrow; plan like you will live forever." A good friend of mine told me this a long time ago, and I've never forgotten it. It made me reflect and realise how very easy it is to let the days of our lives slip through our fingers like grains of sand.

Slowly but surely, life is running out while we tend to live in either the past or the future. Lots of books have been written on the subject, as it's really extremely important to realize that all human beings exist here and now.

Pinch your arm and feel that you're alive

The only time we are really aware of being alive is the nanosecond when we pinch our arm and feel the pain. Everything else is past or present, like a river flowing towards the ocean. It's never ever the same river, even if it looks like it on the surface.

You consist of an exclusive, unique, and enormous mixture of different cells, always changing, always renewing, from the second you were conceived to the day you stop breathing. You are you, but you are definitely not the same you as last year or even last week on a cellular level.

You are renewed, all the time for all of your life

You are constantly being repaired, renewed, and even if you look more or less the same, your cells and body are not. This is the key to rejuvenation; our unique ability to renew, repair, and restore.

It's actually a fact that can change your way of life and make you realize that you can help your body to repair itself to a large degree.

How? By accepting that your cells are constantly making replicas of themselves. If they lack the proper building materials, if they live in a polluted environment, feel starved for oxygen, etc., they will reproduce as best they can, but not as well as they can.

This is very basic biology, and you do not have to be Einstein to realize the consequences. Have a look at this list showing the average time of renewal for different cells. The older you get, the less active you are, the slower the process. But the great thing is that you can, at any time of your life, influence and improve the process.

Renewal time of your cells

You can start pampering the tiny baby cells with the very, very best from nature, and give them the very cleanest and best place to grow and mature. You can feed them with the best and purest foods and fluids and guess you will gradually become a completely NEW YOU, fit to enjoy life at the fullest and looking your very best.

Your skin: 21 to 30 days

Your liver: 42 to 50 days (6 weeks)

Your stomach lining: 5 days

Your DNA: 60 days (2 months)

Your blood: 120 days (4 months)

Your skeleton: 3 months

Your brain: 1 year

Recreate and renew yourself

Everything is based on your DNA - the blueprint of you. The fantastic news is that we can actually influence how our DNA will act when it creates new cells from stem cells. New research has proven that you can actually recreate yourself by improving your lifestyle.

You can turn your inborn characteristics on and off by the thoughts you send them and by your lifestyle. This is scientific fact based on our increasing knowledge of quantum physics, epigenetics, telomeres, and other secrets of cells.

It's actually possible to reprogram, reverse, and repair damage to your DNA and literally experience incredible improvements by using your mind to send the right signals to your body.

You will find the best anti-ageing and rejuvenation techniques that you can do are simple, cheap and available for anybody. It's actually simpler and more basic than you think, and it's very sensible.

It's plain healthy living combined with very positive and problem solving attitude and the ability to relax, enjoy, and appreciate yourself and the people in your life.

I sincerely hope this book will give you the inspiration, motivation, and lots of practical advice so you will succeed in transforming yourself to the best version of you. Take the time you need to remake your lifestyle, yourself, and feel how fantastic it is to be the real you!

Your skin is an indicator of your insides

After a very short period on my lifestyle eating plans and fitness regimes, you will notice changes in your attitude, your body, your mind, and your level of energy. You will certainly start to feel like the master of your universe because you are doing the things that are good for you (even if it takes an effort), which means that you have to say no to lots of temptations.

Your skin will be the first and most visible proof of your internal renewal. You will notice that it gets clearer, brighter, and you actually will have an inner glow.

Follow the daily New You skin and body care routines in this book for three weeks. Give them a real chance, and then you can evaluate the result.

Mirror, mirror on the wall – who is the fairest of them all?

I am convinced that you will say: Mirror, mirror on the wall, I feel fairer than I was... I am on my way! When you make the New You health and beauty regime a regular part of your lifestyle, I'm sure you will be amazed by the results.

You will have to follow the whole plan step by step on a daily basis. It doesn't take long; it doesn't cost much, but it requires that you use a little time and TLC on yourself.

Remember

This book will do nothing for you if you just read it and don't take action. It's a practical book with all you need to rejuvenate yourself. So please give it a chance. Four weeks of your life is a small investment in lifelong health and beauty. This time let the road of good intentions lead to a New You.

Chapter 16

NATURAL SKINCARE

Your skin is the largest organ of your body. It covers 1.5 m2 and this cover is where your life story shows. Everything that happens inside and outside you will reflect on your skin. It's actually true that beauty comes from within. Your skin breathes, absorbs, and gets rid of toxins and dead cells. It's active every second of our lives.

Your skin is a sensory organ, and detects pleasure, pain, lust, temperatures, textures and reflects your feelings instantly. For instance, when you are afraid you get cold, your hair stands up, and you get goose pimples.

Protective cover

Healthy skin protects your organs from damage from your environment, and it's of vital importance that you treat it well. It's the key to your immune defense, as it protects you from dangerous bacteria, virus, fungi, and other harmful substances.

Your skin has the ability to absorb useful - and harmful - substances. This has been known for thousands of years, and remedies have been created to heal, to beautify, to rejuvenate - and also to kill.

Modern pharmacology has invented thousands of synthetic ingredients and combinations that have never before been known to the human race.

The cocktail effect of all these chemicals is seriously dangerous to our health. Many of these chemicals enter our body through our skin and create a multitude of problems, not only with the skin itself, but with our health in general.

Choose natural

I am convinced that it is of vital importance to limit the amount of chemicals we use on our skin for our personal care. I recommend that you are very selective with the ingredients: they should be food grade, as it enters your body via your skin, so this is just as important as the food you eat.

In the chapter DIY Products for Natural Skincare, you will find several very simple yet extremely effective natural products you can make in your own kitchen.

Beauty from within

To keep your skin healthy and as young and supple as possible, it's necessary to feed your skin cells with the right kinds of nutrients: meaning healthy foods and supplements.

Newborn cells (fibroblasts) take three weeks to grow. This means in less than a month your skin is totally new and will reflect what has happened in the last month. Constant stress, lots of toxins, a lack of nutrients and water are examples of a bad start for new cells.

Remember: The cells are constantly being duplicated, and if one generation is undernourished, depleted or mistreated, it will be transferred to the next generation. Visible signs of aging and different skin problems will be the result.

Reverse and repair

The good news is that you can reverse the damage by cleaning up your insides with plenty of good nutrition to give these cells a better start. By detoxing, eating lots of healthy foods, using vitamin and mineral supplements and skincare with natural ingredients, you can totally transform your skin in three to four weeks. I can promise you that the results will astound you. Extra bonus: It will get even better with each passing three-week cell renewal cycle.

Get younger, firmer skin

- Detox inside and outside

- Get plenty of nutrients for growth and repair

- Move and work out to keep your circulation going

- Get enough oxygen

- Drink a minimum of 1.5 litres of water daily

- Sleep 7 - 8 hours a night

- Cleanse, exfoliate, nourish, and hydrate your skin

Facts of life

As we age, our skin thins, bruises more easily, sags and loses much of its firmness and elasticity. That is a fact of life, particularly for women as our estrogen levels drop after the menopause.

Hormone therapy will help to maintain younger, firmer skin, but it might also increase the risk of breast cancer and perhaps other health hazards that we still know little about.

Anti-ageing strategy

To restore a younger, firmer skin we can use several natural products and strategies. In this book, I have focused on "bioceuticals", not pharmaceuticals.

There are certain basic rules to restore sagging skin and renew the quality of skin in general. The underlying structure of the skin is formed of layers of elastin and collagen fibres and subcutaneous fatty deposits combined with muscles that give the skin its shape and form.

If you are too skinny, the skin will be slack and wrinkly and lose its healthy glow. If your diet is lacking in nutrients, the cells will be starved, and it will clearly show when they appear on the surface. They will look old and tired, and so will you!

If you neglect to care for your skin with the right cleansing, stimulation, hydration and supply nutrients from both inside and outside, your skin will reflect it, and you will not be very happy with your mirror image.

If you also neglect the daily pampering of your skin, have taxed it with too much sun, wind, cold, stress and pollution, you will probably have a tough job repairing the lifestyle damages and revert the process.

Seven deadly skin sins

1. Stress and worries

2. Negative attitude

3. Being in the sun without protection

4. Smoking and drug abuse

5. Drinking in excess

6. No cleansing or skincare routine

7. No hydration or nourishing

As you see, this is closely connected with your feelings and attitude. Stress and negativity are very damaging to your skin as well as your general health.

If you have any of the seven problems, try to solve at least some of them. Deep breathing and yoga are natural ways to tackle stress and become more in harmony with yourself.

Skincare rejuvenation program

It's possible for everybody to follow an effective skincare program. It's not particularly expensive (you have a multitude of choices in all price ranges) and it does not require a lot of time. What is required is a bit of know-how, a structured daily treatment and maintenance program, and sticking religiously to it.

Make a covenant with yourself that you will do all it takes to follow all the easy routines for inside and outside for one month.

Use 30 days of your life to restore and improve skin, body, health and energy. When you look in the mirror (and at your before picture), I know you will love the amazing results and the NEW YOU that is gradually emerging from the tired old one.

Your skin covers all of you

Lots of women are good at beauty routines for their face and neck, but they neglect the body care routines that are of vital importance to your total look and wellbeing. Your skin does not end at your neck. It's actually one important organ that covers the whole of YOU, and it's totally connected. That is why you need to treat it from top to toe as it all requires the same daily care and attention as your face.

You need to repair and rejuvenate the whole packaging, making it fresher and glowing again.

New You skincare routine
Cleanse morning and evening

Never go to bed without removing every trace of makeup and dirt that have accumulated during the day. Your pores must be clean so they can breathe freely and absorb the vital ingredients in your night cream.

Exfoliate every other day

Dead cells must be removed from the surface of your skin to keep it glossy and glowing. When you exfoliate and polish your skin, you automatically stimulate the production of collagen and elastin – the elastic fibres that support your skin and keep it young and supple.

Facial with face pack at least twice a week

Pamper your skin with nutrition- filled homemade face packs that make your skin younger, firmer, and with a much younger glow due to increased circulation.

Hydrate and nourish

Look for serums and creams with hyaluronic acid – a natural hydration factor that exists in your body. The higher the level of hyaluronic acid, the more your cells plump up with water. The difference can be amazing, like the difference between a grape and a raisin.

Look for products with antioxidants and natural vegetable oils. Avoid products with mineral oils and synthetic ingredients.

Use sunscreen and protect your skin

I live on an island with sun all year round, but I avoid baking in the sun. I use thin kaftans and big sun hats for protection to avoid having to use synthetic creams. If and when I relax on a sun bed, I am always protected by a parasol.

Lots of sunscreens are totally synthetic, so it's not easy to protect in a natural way. I use Aloe Vera sun lotion. It's also fantastic as an after-sun cooler and skin restorer.

I also use natural yoghurt as an after sun, as it's one of the oldest and best remedies for your skin. It's a lifesaver if you should get sunburn.

Avoid dangerous D deficiency

It's important to get some sun on unprotected skin so your skin can produce enough of the important sunshine vitamin D. Increased deficiencies have been observed in recent years, most likely a result of the increased use of sunscreens.

It's very, very dangerous for our health, because recent research has shown that vitamin D is the on-and-off trigger for our immune defense system, so you can end up with some dangerous illnesses and health troubles if you are lacking this super important vitamin.

Make your own natural beauty products

Are you getting more and more skeptical about all the manmade ingredients we use in food, cosmetics, clothes, and virtually most things that we use in our everyday consumer society? Do you feel that we are on a dangerous, destructive path against nature?

What you put on your body is absorbed by the skin and transported deep into your organism. We know little about the long-term effect of all these" magical" synthetic ingredients. How they interact and influence our DNA is anybody's guess.

If you seriously want to reduce your use of harmful products and find more natural and healthier alternatives, I will share my very simple products with you. They are all from the kitchen cupboard and they are used for cooking as well as personal care. In other words, they are good enough – and safe enough – to eat.

Forget the glossy, super expensive products that are decorating your bathroom shelf. Put them away for three weeks. Go natural and see what happens when the newborn skin cells come to the surface in just three to four weeks.

Chapter 17

DIY PRODUCTS FOR NATURAL SKINCARE

A good vegetable oil

Cleansing your skin every evening to you get rid of all dirt, pollution and makeup is a must for skin health. In the morning it's usually enough to rinse your face in lukewarm water and finish with ice cold to close your pores, or just stand under the shower and let it do the job while you wake up.

A cold pressed, good quality virgin oil is my favourite product for cleansing. It's a super makeup remover and dissolves even long lasting and waterproof mascara.

Oils make the skin soft, supple, and increase its ability to stay hydrated. It also strengthens the acid balance, which is very important for your whole immune system. Olive oil, avocado oil, grape seed oil, sunflower oil, or coconut oil are all excellent for skincare. Try them out and find what is best for you. Grape seed and sunflower are very neutral and don´t smell oily and they are very good combined with essential oils.

Goodbye plastic, hello glass

If you really want to go green, stop buying products in plastic packaging. I use glass bottles with cork stoppers for my oils, and small glass jars for gels and other of my home-made products. It's very pretty packaging, and free of logos and stickers. You can glam them up with silk ribbons too.

Peeling without plastic

Regular peeling is very important for skin health and for a youthful look. Peeling stimulates the skin cells and kicks them into action, so they increase their production of collagen and elastine.

Unfortunately, most peelings contain plastic micro beads that are seriously dangerous to nature, animals, and humans. The particles are so small that they are actually being absorbed by our body. We must avoid this all cost and natural alternatives.

Brushes are great

Use them to polish your face in up and outward circles. Use bigger ones to brush your body. You can do this on a daily basis to increase circulation and get a healthy glow as well as improved texture.

Polish your skin with sugar

Mix one cup of olive oil or cocoa butter with 2 cups of coarse brown sugar. Add a few drops of lemon and stir it all to an even paste. Pour it into a glass jar with a tight lid (old jam jars are perfect). Clean your skin.

Take a little paste and peel with up and outward circular movements. Be extra meticulous on the T-zone where the pores tend to be more clogged. Remove with sponges and rinse, rinse, rinse. Finish with ice cold running water, and massage Aloe Vera gel into your skin.

Pineapple Enzymatic Peeling

Pineapple contains an enzyme that dissolves dead skin cells, and it's a great alternative to use for peeling. Cut a big slice of fresh pineapple, remove the skin, and cut into small pieces. Crush and blend it to an even paste. Add rice flour, corn flour or potato flour so the paste gets stickier and is easier to use.

First clean your skin and rub it well with a fresh piece of pineapple. Then put on the face pack in an even layer. Use a brush if you need to. If you have coarse, sun damaged or wrinkly skin, leave it for 20 minutes. If you have thin, sensitive skin with red spider veins, leave it on for 10 minutes to start with.

Improve and pamper your skin with face packs

You can use most fruits and berries to make wonderful face masks. Just mash them into an even pulp, drain off extra fluid, and add some oil and rice flour to give it a creamier texture that is easy to use. You can also use white clay as a base, which you can get for next to nothing at most chemists.

Baking Soda

This is so versatile, easy to use, natural, very cheap, and absolutely one product you need for everything in your green life. It's great for skin and body care, for your brilliant white smile, for killing germs and fungi, and even for more or less all cleaning jobs around the house – from your oven and toilet, to tiles and crystal glasses.

In the bathroom, baking soda is perfect for easy peeling of face and body, for brushing and whitening your teeth, strengthening your gums, and killing germs, and is anti-bacterial and anti-fungal so it helps with feet too.

The secrets of Elizabeth Arden's beauty salon in London

My first source of inspiration to fruity, natural masks was after I interviewed celebrity designers and makeup artists in London, in addition to hunting for news from the most famous beauty salons.

I chose Elizabeth Arden and made an appointment for a facial behind their famous red door….

I wanted to know what they were using and recommending. In additions to their brand name cleansers and creams, they used natural face masks and remedies they made themselves in a room behind the treatment rooms.

After my treatment (a very good one, I might add), I was allowed in on their secret.

The manageress was a lady in her late sixties with beautiful, natural, and seemingly ageless skin. She confessed that natural remedies were one of her secrets, and that was why they used them for their famous beauty treatments. This has always inspired me, and I hope it will inspire you. Here are some of my skin food goodies. Mix, mash, and pamper yourself the natural way.

Go bananas

Ripe bananas are so rich in minerals, vitamins, and nutrients, plus they are the most perfect meal in their own package. They are perfect skin food too. Crush and blend a banana into an even paste. Add some oil if your skin is dry and apply.

Egg yolk is wonderful for dry skin

You can mix an egg yolk with a little rice or corn flour for a creamy, nutritious mask that is loaded with beneficial fatty acids. This is just the thing for a dry and ageing skin. You can even add extra oil, so just experiment.

Avocado is extremely rejuvenating and anti-wrinkle

Avocado is my favourite, and the puree you make from it is a Cinderella treatment for dry, tired, dehydrated, and wrinkled skin. The essential fatty acids make your skin softer, more elastic, and full of moisture.

Take the meat from half an avocado and mash it until creamy. You can add some oil and rice flour to make it more solid.

Clean and peel your skin and put on thick layer on your face, neck and décolleté. Relax for 30 minutes before you rinse it off. You will love the result.

Hydrating Aloe Vera

Use pure, organic Aloe Vera Gel in an even layer on clean skin. You can use it daily if you need too. The Aloe Vera gel improves and heals skin damage and makes your skin healthier, younger looking, and more elastic. It also improves the protective acid layer of your skin. You can use the gel as your daily moisturizer for face and body. You will love the results.

The all-round natural green soap

Natural, fluid soap (green soap or castile soap) has been used forever for everything from cleaning your home to your face and body, and hair washing. It's an unbeatable remedy for sore, scaly feet and hard skin. It's also simple, cheap and quite natural.

You can add your favourite essential oil to the castile soap and make your special signature shower gels and shampoos to save money and the environment.

Apply moisturizing hair and face mask

Moisten your hair by massaging in honey mixed with an egg yolk. The same mixture can be used as a face mask. Feel free to add oats to make it firmer. This is an incredibly moisturizing and refreshing treatment for both skin and hair.

You should leave the mask on for at least 15 minutes, so relax and enjoy the experience while daydreaming and having a full timeout. Why not place cold cucumber slices on the eye area for a firming and refreshing effect and to reduces swelling.

Remove the mask with hot flannels and plenty of water. Wash your hair with glycerin soap or mild, natural shampoo at least twice. Massage the scalp well. Rinse well and add some vinegar in the last rinse water for extra shine. If you are blonde, then lemon or chamomile is great in the final rinse.

Vinegar balances the pH value of your skin

Vinegar contains antioxidants that fight free radicals, bacteria and fungi. It has an acidic pH value, and it therefore helps restore the skin's protective acid mantle. You can also mix vinegar with water in a jug and use it as a rinse to make your hair extra shiny.

Natural anti-ageing skin serum

The small beauty capsules from the famous cosmetic brands cost a small fortune. They are loaded with promises and "secret" ingredients. Try this natural alternative instead, and I promise you it's really super food for your skin.

These are natural vitamin E capsules that you buy in the health food store filled with pure vitamin E. Pinch a hole in a capsule, and massage the serum into your clean skin before you go to bed. This is superb as a rejuvenating serum and contains effective antioxidants that protect the skin.

Sparkly clean makeup brushes and sponges

Clean your makeup brushes and sponges regularly to avoid a build- up of makeup residue and bacteria. I like to use some olive oil with a dash of castile soap! It gives super clean soft brushes, which gives a smooth and even makeup application.

DIY saves nature and improves your skin health

You can save money on switching to natural products you make yourself, and you can save yourself and nature a lot of unnecessary synthetics. If we all make our little effort, it will contribute to a cleaner environment.

Essential oils and aromatherapy

The wonderful concentrated drops from plants and flowers have extreme therapeutic value. They have been part of natural medicine for thousands of years, and they are the components of the classic perfumes and organic, natural cosmetics.

Unfortunately, a lot of synthetic copies are used today. They have the aroma, but not the effect on your nervous system, your feelings, or your skin and body health.

You can easily get all the fantastic effects by learning to use quality essential aromatic oils to your benefit. Start off with a few all-purpose oils and then you can expand when you have more experience. It's so easy to start with.

Fill a small glass bottle with a cold pressed virgin vegetable oil of your choice. Add a few drops of your favourite essential oil that is suitable for your type of skin.

Essential, safe oils

Here are the oils that you can easily use at home. They have delicious scents, wonderfully good effects, and are very suitable when making your own natural cosmetics. Because the oils have hundreds of components, they also have a large treatment area. Here are just a few of the properties of the oils I recommend for home and natural cosmetics.

- Lavender. Playful, deodorizing, nerve-relaxing, harmonizing, soothing

- Sweet orange. Against fatigue and general weariness

- Neroli, orange blossom. Curbs anxiety, extremely calming

- Frankincense, incense. Very soothing and puts one in a spiritual mood

- Rose: Rejuvenating for the skin and comforting

- Peppermint. Invigorating

- Rosemary. Rejuvenating

- Clementine. New energy

- Sandalwood. Harmonizing, aphrodisiac

- Cinnamon. Warming, anti-bacterial

- Ylang-ylang. Balancing, aphrodisiac

- Cedar. Anti-stress, aphrodisiac

- Chamomile. Calming

- Lemon. Firming

- Eucalyptus. Facilitates breathing and improves respiratory infections

- Geranium. Revitalizing, hormone balancing for women

- Basil. Stimulating, provides clearer brain and concentration

- Tea Tree. Antiseptic, anti-bacterial, anti-fungal and anti-viral. A natural alternative to antibiotics

- Petit Grain. Anti-depressant

- Patchouli. Regenerating

- Rosewood. Encouraging

- Grapefruit. Refreshing, stimulating

Did you know?

- Some essential oils are more expensive than gold per gram

- It takes tons of rose petals to make a bottle of extract

- The quality and the forces depend on the polluted growing place

- Men associate the scent of vanilla with breasts

- The oil clary sage makes you feel both lively and relaxed

- Orange flowers and neroli curb anxiety

- Ylang-ylang is a powerful aphrodisiac

- Ginger is the world's best remedy for seasickness and nausea

- Chamomile provides immediate relief to troubled colic children

- Tea tree is natural antibiotic that also works against fungi and viruses

- A drop of sandalwood behind the ear makes you a man magnet

Synthetic copies may have identical scents, but they have none of these beneficial properties and do not affect the parasympathetic nervous system. Therefore, synthetic perfumes have no sensual, attractive or natural medicinal value.

The first genuine ones that I recommend to most people are precious and very therapeutic: Geranium, lavender and orange flower. I also recommend Eucalyptus for clearing the nose and airways.

Use your nose and sniff around when you are in the health food store and ask for advice and recommendations. Their staff often have a high level of expertise and experience.

Chapter 18

NUTRITION FOR A NEW YOU

If you want to improve your health, energy, skin quality and reduce your biological age, changing your eating habits is the most important step to a New You. All you need is to combine natural, nutrition-packed foods and drinks with enough physical activity. Add on enough sleep, a positive attitude, proper skin and body care, and you will shed years.

Don't fall for fads

Because nutrition is a complex field with often contradictory information, it's vital to understand the undisputed basics. Forget all the miracle cures and fad diets because they won't work in the long run. If they did, we would all be slim and healthy.

My best advice to you is to forget the fads, forget empty promises, and stick to what has worked for the human race for thousands of years: Natural, unprocessed foods in limited quantities according to your size and level of activity.

Don't stuff yourself

To make it easy, you can visualize a normal – not too big – dinner plate, and divide it into three sections: 40 %, 40 % and 20 %. Fill one of the sections with protein-rich food, the other with vegetables, and the third with complex carbohydrates like rice, potatoes, etc.

Why? These three main nutrients are the components of all foods and drinks on this planet, and we need all of them in different quantities according to our size, gender, activity level, biochemical identity and metabolism, lifestyle and stress level.

You have to find out how much food/ calories your body needs to stay healthy. You have to establish how much you can eat when you need to lose weight, and how much you can eat when you want to maintain your ideal weight.

Facts about Nutrition

You probably know quite a lot about the different nutrients and their importance for your body chemistry, but I think repeating it here will do you no harm. It's quite smart to learn a bit more about nutrition to really understand the importance of getting what your body needs to stay in perfect health.

When you fill your body with everything it needs, it has an amazing ability to stay healthy, fight off intruders like bacteria, virus, fungi etc., and repair any damages.

Without the necessary nutrients, it's very difficult for your body to cope. Though your body can survive a lot of abuse and malnourishment, in the end, it starts to malfunction. Result: The body shows more and more symptoms and minor ailments that gradually manifest as illnesses.

A well-balanced diet with enough nutrients is the foundation of health, wellbeing, energy, and good looks. It's the most important preventive medicine and anti-ageing cure. So, take your time to learn more about it and even if you have pretty good knowledge of the subject, it's smart to stay updated.

Protein 1 gram is 4 kcal

Without protein, there is no life! To repair and renew the cells of your body requires enough complete protein to produce all the necessary amino acids that are the building blocks of your whole body.

Animal protein is a complete source. The safest and easiest way to cover your needs is to choose fish, fowl, meat, eggs, and dairy products.

If you are a vegetarian, it's a bit more complicated, as vegetarian protein is incomplete and has to be combined in a very special way to make it possible for the body to produce the vital amino acids. If you are a vegetarian, you can use beans, lentils, and similar sources of vegetable proteins combined with bread and dairy products.

Enough protein is a must for growth and repair

It's very important to know that getting enough protein is crucial to delay the ageing process and keep you fit, healthy, and attractive. If you get too little protein (less than 1 gram per kg bodyweight per day), your body will increase the percentage of fatty tissue as it literally steals protein from your muscles and lean body tissues to cover the need for amino acids. This is a sheer survival response of your body to keep your cells alive.

Protein deficiency reduces the production of glucagon, the important fat-burning hormone. This means that low protein intake will make you fatter and wobblier.

It will also lead to rapidly ageing skin with sagging and wrinkles, as your body lacks enough building material to repair the collagen and elastin fibres that keep your skin firm and elastic.

High protein low carb diets

The older you get, the more proteins you need for the body to repair and rebuild itself. But the intake should be within sensible limits, and from good quality sources like meat, fish, fowl, and eggs.

Restricted intake of all refined carbs is sensible for everybody, but to reduce carb intake to such a minimum that you get into a state of ketosis is not such a good idea. It can be downright dangerous and unhealthy.

Such restricted diets can be good for a short period for those with diabetes and serious obesity, but it should be followed up by a doctor who is nutrition oriented. For others a mixed diet is advised.

Don't fool yourself

One reason why low carb diets seem to work like a charm at the start is that they are diuretic. This means that you lose a lot of water, and it shows on the scales. The problem is that most protein diets are high in calories too as they allow you to eat lots of fatty foods. They are difficult to stick to long term as so many foods and drinks are prohibited.

When you fall off the high protein-low carb wagon (as everybody does after a short while of unsocial, unbalanced eating), you are likely to add on more weight than you lost. Then welcome to the worldwide club of yo-yo dieters who are slimming themselves fat...

Fat: 1 gram is 9 kcal

Humans need fats, so fat-free diets are very unhealthy. We have several types of fat, and we need a little bit of each to ensure that we produce the fatty acids necessary for many metabolic processes.

It's important as a lubricant, for the health and look of your skin, all the membranes in your body, for your nerves and nerve endings – the signal transmitters of your brain and for the absorption of fat-soluble vitamins, just to mention some of the vital purposes of fat in a daily diet.

Animal fat

Foods that are high in protein normally contain a certain percentage of animal fat. Too much is bad for you, but a little is good because your body needs a lot of different fatty acids to function properly.

Omega 3 oil from fish fat, particularly salmon, is fantastic; it gives you younger, more glowing and supple skin as well as protecting your cardiovascular system. It's the number one preventive medicine for heart disease.

As one gram of fat provides 9 kcal of energy, it's important to remove visible fat from meat.

Vegetable fat

Vegetables contain important fatty acids that are a must for your health and beauty. Grains, seeds and nuts are prime sources of the vital anti-ageing vitamin E (a precursor of Q10), which is a potent cell protector that inhibits attacks from dangerous free oxygen radicals that can alter their properties and turn malignant.

Olive oil is the most treasured source, so please enjoy a daily dose. However, buy a prime quality virgin oil that is cold pressed, and avoid plant oils that are heat processed or transformed to trans-fat. Those are sheer poison for your body and can seriously damage your health. Heat treated vegetable oils change from healthy to dangerous because they contain many dangerous free oxygen radicals.

Stay away from all kinds of deep-fried foods and fast foods. Can you imagine the unhealthy oil filled with dangerous free radicals that they use in the fast food places? How often do they change it?

Trans fat is dangerous

This is a fat based on vegetable oils, but chemically altered to suit the needs of the food industry as an amalgamator, taste enhancer, and a cheap substitute for butter and natural fats. Because it's based on vegetable oils, the advertising and packaging claims it's good for you – and it's a great big lie.

Why? It's a man-made product where the plant oils are altered in a way that can lead to serious degeneration of our bodies because we lack the enzymes to break it down and metabolize it.

Trans fats are prohibited in Denmark and more countries are following, but it takes time to eliminate this health hazard because of the enormous economic consequences. You can eat smart and avoid it like the plague it is.

Beware that "healthy, heart friendly" soy margarine is also a man-made product with heaps of trans fat manufactured from soy oil – more often than not made from genetically altered soybeans. No one knows the consequences consuming it will have on our bodies and genetic material.

Carbohydrates 1 gram is 4 kcal

On and on, they are your best friend, but they can also be your lethal enemy. You certainly know that low-carb or no-carb diets have been the answer to the prayers of hopeful slimmer's.

An enormous industry of prefabricated low-carb foods and drinks is the result, and it has turned in to a multibillion-dollar business.

And guess what: The average weight of people in the Western world is increasing to an all-time high, causing the World Health Organization (WHO) to brand this as our major health challenge of the century.

So, obviously, the light products and sweeteners does not work. The reason is pretty simple: a lack of understanding of how the different foods, drinks and prefab, industrial foods with lots of chemicals affect our intricate body chemistry.

To brand carbs as the enemy is wrong, it is the refined sugar and flour that should be avoided! The complex carbohydrates should be eaten in much bigger quantities. We should go much greener, and we would improve our health and wellbeing and get slimmer at the same time.

The clue lies in the two different main groups of carbohydrates: refined and natural.

Complex carbohydrates: Starches

Vegetables, fruits, berries, grains, and nuts are our sources of carbohydrates needed for sufficient energy to keep us going. In their natural state, they contain loads of vitamins, minerals, roughage, fruit sugars, and important micronutrients. As one gram represents only 4 kcal of energy, you can eat large quantities and fill your stomach without getting fat. It's prime fuel for your cells!

Refined carbs are ruined carbs

The refining process removes a lot – or all – of the nutrients, and you end up with second rate fuel that provides nothing more than energy (i.e. calories). Sugar is an excellent example of the complexity of this biochemical fact. Sugar cane in its natural state is a big part of the staple diet in sugar-producing countries.

It baffled the scientists that the workers had virtually no cavities and the most brilliant, strong teeth. How could that be? Everybody knew that sugar was number one tooth enemy, leading to decay and rot.

Finnish scientists found the answer in a substance in non-processed sugar cane, and they gave it the magic name Xylitol. This is probably the most potent cavity-preventing element in the world, and today you find it everywhere: for example, in chewing gum.

We think we are smart, but nature is smarter. It can be complicated to understand why, because so many biological ingredients are still to be discovered, so we have to trust what has been tried, used and appreciated for eons by humans, and are still in use.

Facts of your daily bread

Grains have been a staple food of the human diet from our early history. They are the source of energy, of vegetable proteins, roughage, of vital minerals and vitamins, particularly vitamin B complex and vitamin E.

It's a very sad fact that this main nutrient source has been gradually ruined, refined, and robbed of more or less all-natural nutrients. The outer layers of the grains are removed in the milling process, and what is left is a kernel containing carbohydrates that have no nutritional value – only calories.

A lot of the grains are also genetically "improved", meaning that we really do not know the consequences to our health. Most of this is industrial white flour and products made from it. No wonder that gluten allergies and lots of other food allergies are spreading like wildfire.

The manipulated foods robbed of nutrients are dangerous to our health, and the only way to protect yourself is to be eat as many natural and unrefined foods as possible.

White sugar is a health hazard

My best health and beauty advice is to avoid refined carbohydrates and all kinds of foods that are loaded with white sugar and white flour. Go for the real things as much as possible. You will find most of what you need in ordinary supermarkets, so it's fairly easy to avoid the sugar trap.

Beware of the declarations on the packaging as there is no distinction between refined and unrefined carbohydrates. You have to be your own nutrition expert to improve your health and avoid the traps. The good news is that it's very easy once you know the difference.

Stay healthy with Lifestyle Medicine

An active lifestyle will prevent a lot of serious diseases, from heart problems, to auto-immune diseases, cancers etc. The wrong lifestyle has created a worldwide tsunami of diabetes and high blood pressure.

It's killing so many nutrition illiterate people or ruining their quality of life from an early age. You can avoid being a victim, and you can turn the tide if you already have problems.

My lifestyle medicine is one that you will enjoy because the only side effects are a better body, better health and better looks. Healthy, natural foods are the best medicine with no side effects. Those who would suffer most would be the global pharmaceutical companies and industrial food processors.

Alcohol: 1 gram is 7 kcal

Alcohol contains calories that can be a substantial part of daily intake if you drink too much. The sweeter the drinks, the more calories they contain. A modest intake of wine is considered good for you, as it will make you feel good, relaxed, and improve your digestion. It will also be beneficial for your heart, as it makes the blood "thinner" and improves circulation in general.

Red wine contains reservatrol, an anti-aging component that is extremely valuable for keeping us young and healthy. White wine is produced by skinned grapes, so it does not contain this ingredient that is part of the grape skin.

Wines are fermented fruits and vegetables, and contain a lot of good nutrients, but beware of the negative aspects as well.

Alcohol is metabolized differently from foods, and it all happens in the liver. That is why the over-consumption or abuse of alcohol gradually leads to liver problems.

Alcohol is also very dehydrating, so when you drink it, always supply your body with the same amount of water to counteract dehydration. There is also a toll on your kidneys, so flush them and clean them with loads of water and add some lemon to enhance the elimination process.

You should avoid drinking alcohol when you want to lose weight or limit it to only a couple of glasses of dry wine once in a while.

Coffee and tea

Our favourite drinks contain no calories, but they can have other beneficial effects on your body if they are not chemically tampered with. Coffee is a diuretic, so you should drink a minimum of equal amounts of water when you enjoy it.

An espresso is so condensed and strong that you need a big glass of water as a chaser. Coffee is considered good for you as long as you make it properly from good quality organic beans. Make it the Mediterranean way, not in a percolator.

You are 60% water

Your body is literally filled with water! A newborn baby can contain as much as 75% water, but this decreases gradually with age. In an adult, nearly 60% – more than half of your body weight – is water.

However, these are averages and will vary according to body composition and gender. Overweight individuals have a significantly lower level, sometimes as low as 45%.

The water level of your body is regulated by anti-diuretic hormones and a special peptide to maintain safe levels. It's vital to drink enough water to keep these normal levels, and particularly during strenuous exercise, sweating, hot weather, and dry indoor climates, it's crucial to get enough water or diuretic drinks to prevent illnesses like diarrhea, vomiting, and fever. The other option is to supply your body with enough water-soluble vitamins and minerals to replace what is lost.

Beware of dehydration

Loss of fluids can cause dehydration, potassium deficiency, salt imbalances, and seriously lower the levels of electrolytes. A potassium and/or magnesium deficiency is extremely dangerous, as it can lead to palpitations and irregular heartbeats and cardiac arrest as a worst-case scenario.

My guess is that this is the reason why quite a number of athletes and fitness addicts develop heart problems. There is nothing wrong with their heart; they are just being deprived of minerals and electrolytes due to extreme dehydration and water loss over time, so their body stores are virtually empty.

The safest way is daily supplements and to use natural mineral water as your daily drinking water. This is extremely important if your tap water is recycled and tampered with, like in most urban areas.

Chapter 19

LIFE DEPENDS ON VITAMINS AND MINERALS

Micronutrients are the pillars of all the intricate metabolic functions and interactions of your body. There is serious synergy, but we still have a lot to discover in this enormous field of biology and biochemistry. But a few vital points about what is considered essential to life are interesting for you and I would like to share them.

The following pages are a crash course on the different vitamins and minerals. It's particularly useful for you to read about the many health problems that occur when the body is depleted of these vital nutrients. In fact, much of what we know as illnesses is really quite simply serious malnutrition.

Fat- and water-soluble vitamins

There are two different kinds of vitamins: water soluble or fat soluble. Water soluble vitamins are not stored for a long time in your body and so must be replaced according to how much your body uses. This will depend a lot on your lifestyle, level of stress, pollution, eating and drinking habits, body composition, and genetic inheritance.

Fat soluble vitamins are stored in your body, and it takes time to deplete the stores, but they are as important.

Get enough to stay healthy

A good piece of advice is it to maintain your vitamin levels by eating well, adjusting to your needs, and taking enough supplements to counteract the lack of nutrients in industrialized foods.

Mass production, transport, storage, the need for long shelf life, competitive prices, and attractive foods have seriously affected the level of vitamins and minerals in most foods. We need to make wise choices in our choice of foods.

Modern, industrialized foods are less risky when it comes to bacteria, fungi, and other elements that can make us sick, so we have to take the sweet with the sour and add to what our modern, hygienic foods lack into our own diets.

Fatty acids and oils Vegetable Oils

Plant oils from avocado, wheat germ, coconut, apricot, grape seed, jojoba, almonds, hazelnuts, and other nuts contain different beneficial fatty acids for a healthy skin. They are excellent as rejuvenators, and recommended for regular massage as they improve elasticity, firmness, and prevent dehydration. Oils with high levels of gamma linoleic acid (GLA) are particularly healing for sensitive, dehydrated, itchy, scaling skins with eczema and similar problems. They are used as food supplements and for external use (like a serum).

My daily supplements: For more than 40 years, I have more or less used the highest doses of multivitamin minerals and mega doses (1 to 5 grams) of Vitamin C (ascorbic acid) daily.

The more stress I feel or with any risk of infectious diseases like flu etc., I take larger doses. Very stressful periods can also require higher doses of the B-complex. I also take 400 IU of fat-soluble vitamin E (the recommended daily amount in International Units). In periods I also take extra Magnesium,

We are all very different, and we all have different needs, but I advise you to try this complete regime for a month.

Chapter 20

FAT SOLUBLE VITAMINS

Fat soluble vitamins are stored in your body in reasonable quantities. This means you can get by for a while even if you get too little in your daily food. But the more we learn about these vitamins, the more important they seem to be for a multitude of biochemical functions.

Vitamin A

This is extremely important for your skin, your skin colour, your membranes, eyesight, and growth in general. If you have poor night vision, skin problems or a dry feeling inside your nostrils, these are a few indications of low levels.

- *Vitamin A is important for:*

- *The quality and look of your skin*

- *Elasticity and rejuvenation of cells*

- *All mucus membranes*

- *Normal cell growth*

- *Transferring light impulses to your visual nerves*

- *Your immune defenses (the skin's acid mantle protects against invaders)*

- *General health*

- *Feedback from the environment*

- *Pain and pleasure signals*

- *Temperature regulation*

Lack of Vitamin A can lead to:

- *Premature ageing, sagging skin, and wrinkles*

- *Age spots, pigmentation problems.*

- *Scaly, dry, dehydrated skin*

- *Infections in the mucus membranes and airways*

- *Stunted growth in childhood*

- *Loss of night vision*

- *Eye problems and eye diseases*

If you have damaged skin with premature wrinkles, sagging and spots, I recommend that you visit your doctor and get a prescription for Vitamin A cream. It can do wonders for restoring your skin.

The first treatment period can be rather uncomfortable as your skin will get red and painful as dead cells are shed. But gradually the skin gets used to it and becomes stronger, producing younger cells so you will look years younger. Don't forget to use sunscreen every day too.

Vitamin D

This is a pro-vitamin known as the sunshine vitamin, as it's produced in your own skin when the thin layer of sebum covering it is exposed to sun and daylight. Other sources are from foods like fish and dairy products.

Vitamin D is extremely important for your immune system and many other processes in your body. If you lack Vitamin D, your body cannot absorb calcium. In children, this can lead to rickets; in adults it will lead to osteoporosis, an all too common, disabling disease. This is partly due to the survival mechanism of your body.

When deprived of calcium due to a Vitamin D-induced lack of absorption, your body will literally steal calcium from your bones and teeth in order to get enough calcium to maintain the transfer of nerve signals to keep you alive. This includes the nerve signals needed to keep your heart beating.

Just as important as strong bones is a strong immune defense system and new research has proven that sufficient vitamin D is vital to turn on the immune functions. If you have a deficiency, you leave your body open to all kinds of infection and diseases. A word of warning: an increasing Vitamin D deficiency is occurring in the wake of our increased use of sunscreen to protect us from skin cancer and wrinkles. If you expose your skin to sun for at least 15 minutes before you put on your sunscreen or sun lotion, your skin will manage to absorb enough of this vital vitamin. You can of course protect your sensitive face and neck but let the rest of your body enjoy the precious sunshine to fill your Vitamin D stores to the brim.

It's very important for coloured people living in northern Europe to remember to take adequate Vitamin D supplements as their skin is genetically different and needs lots of sunshine to produce enough. For babies and children, it's a must to avoid rickets!!

Vitamin D is Important for:

- *Absorption of calcium and phosphorus in the intestine*

- *Enough calcium for strong and healthy teeth and bones*

- *Transferring nerve impulses*

Lack of Vitamin D can lead to:

- *Osteoporosis*

- *Cavities and teeth problems*

- *Rickets*

- *Muscle cramps - including irregular heart rhythm*

It can also lead to weakened immune defense, making you less resistant to all kind of infections and illnesses.

Vitamin E

This vitamin is extremely important for your cells, your skin, your energy, and immune defenses. It's also the best anti-ageing component you can add to your diet.

It has been proven in a multitude of scientific studies that a daily dose of 400 IU of Vitamin E prevents all kinds of cardiovascular diseases, so it's the number one heart protector.

It was called the sex vitamin among biochemists, as it leads to more energy. Earlier studies have also shown that it can be very beneficial for couples who have fertility problems. Unfortunately, this lacks definitive evidence as vitamin therapy is not a very lucrative niche in the pharmaceutical market.

Vitamin E improves the circulation and is a natural blood thinner/ anti-coagulant. It's so effective that plastic surgeons always ask their patients to cut it out before operations.

Vitamin E also greatly improves the body's ability to utilize oxygen, so it's great for anybody with respiratory problems and grey, dull skin.

If you ever go to the Andes or other extremely high-altitude areas where breathing is difficult, Vitamin E is the key to use whatever oxygen is available and so you can breathe more easily. This, combined with strong black coffee, is the survival trick from Europeans who have worked there. Indigenous people chew marihuana leaves, and those in the Andes chew cocoa for the same effect, which just proves that sometimes nature is way ahead of us.

Vitamin E supplements are also fantastic for people with sun sensitive skin and prickly heat problems, as well as for normalizing sebum production that results in acne and skin problems in general. It's also great for improving scars, stretch marks, and wrinkles. It's a great first aid solution for burns, and skin healing without scarring. Keep capsules with fluid Vitamin E in the house in case of serious burns. Dab it immediately on dry skin after cooling the affected area under lots of cold running water. You can also use the content of the capsules as a super anti-ageing serum under your normal creams.

Vitamin E is important for:

- *Building and restoring muscle mass*

- *Youthful, firm, elastic skin*

- *Fertility*

- *Hormone production*

- *Normal cell growth*

- *Liver function*

- *Fat metabolism*

- *Protects Vitamin A and fatty acids from free-radical attacks and oxidizing*

- *Utilization of oxygen*

Lack of Vitamin E can lead to:

- *Anaemia*

- *Reduced muscle strength*

- *Hormonal problems*

- *Ulcers that heal slowly*

- *Heart and circulation problems*

- *Sun sensitivity, skin allergies*

- *Premature ageing*

- *Inability to conceive*

Vitamin K

This fat-soluble vitamin is a member of a group of similar, less known vitamins that are vital for normal blood coagulation. They also play different roles in complicated metabolic processes in bone and other tissue.

Traditionally, supplements have not been recommended, as nutritionists thought that the good bacteria in your gut produce sufficient amounts of K.

However, in the last few years, more and more research has shown that the Vitamin K, particularly K2, is very important for a healthy heart.

It's also important to remember that antibiotics and different medicines can seriously damage the natural production of useful bacteria in your body. This means that you will need probiotics to restore the normal balance, and probably extra supplements.

The good news is that green leafy vegetables are a super source, as the K vitamin systems are actually the human body's version of plant photosynthesis. Again, food is your medicine.

Vitamin K is important for:

- *Normal coagulation of the blood*

- *Possibly for healthy heart functions*

Lack of Vitamin K can lead to:

- *Stroke*

- *Issues in new borns*

Chapter 21

WATER-SOLUBLE VITAMINS

These vitamins are unfortunately not stored in significant quantities in the body. They must be supplied preferably on a daily basis, and it's extremely important to increase your intake during stress, pollution, illnesses, and while taking medication.

A lack of water-soluble vitamins can have very serious consequences for mental and physical health, and also for the efficiency of the immune system.

Vitamin C

This water-soluble vitamin is also part of a complex. It's an antioxidant, and perhaps the most vital component of a functioning, strong immune system. If you have any kind of infection or inflammation, it works faster than any antibiotic I know. The storage capacity of the body for this critical life vitamin is very limited, and you burn it off in no time if you are unwell.

Vitamin C is involved in a multitude of complex metabolic processes, and it affects all your connective tissues, your production of collagen, cell membranes, hormones, and immune defenses. It strengthens the capillaries and the viscosity of your blood as it acts as a natural thinner. It also improves the absorption of iron.

Visible signs of low levels of Vitamin C are bruising, constant inflammation – like acne – and all kinds of infections from sore throat to common colds and respiratory problems.

The daily dose will vary from person to person and from day to day, all depending on stress, pollution, use of medicines, and a multitude of other lifestyle factors. To test if your stores are filled, you must try it out. Start with a gram of pure Vitamin C and take several at two-hour intervals during the day. A touch of diahorrea indicates your body stores are full, so you can reduce the intake.

Vitamin B Complex

This is a group consisting of many different vitamins with different properties and metabolic functions. Because they all work together in complicated processes in your body, they will all affect your physical and mental health in a multitude of ways.

If you overdose on one of them for a period, you can have a deficiency in the others, so you should take them all in the correct interactive doses.

The B team is in abundance in most foods and drinks, from animal and plant sources, and it would take too long to go through them all, but here are the main ones.

B1 (Thiamin) Important for:

- *The carbohydrate metabolism*

- *Transferring nerve impulses*

- *Stamina*

- *Digestion*

Lack of B1 can lead to:

- *Beri-Beri*

- *Lack of appetite*

- *Obstipation*

- *Nervousness*

- *Depression*

- *Insomnia and sleep problems*

- *Weakness of the heart function*

- *Muscle pains*

- *Muscle cramps*

B2 (Riboflavin) Important for:

- *Normal metabolism*

- *Skin and mucus membranes*

- *Vision and functioning of the eyes*

Lack of B2 can lead to:

- *Sores and cracks around eyes, ears, and mouth*

- *Scaly facial skin, irritations, and spots*

- *Burning, tired eyes*

- *Dry throat and problems swallowing*

- *Digestive problems*

B3 (Niacinamid) Important for:

- *Carbohydrate metabolism*

- *Normal functions of the skin and mucus membranes*

- *The nervous system*

Lack of B3 can lead to:

- *Pellagra skin disease*

- *Lack of appetite*

- *Sickness and diarrhorea*

- *Dark pigmentation spots on face and neck*

- *Scaly, uneven, rough skin*

- *Sore, red tongue*

- *Nerve pains*

- *Headache*

- *Dizziness*

- *Depression*

B5 (Pantothenic Acid) Important for:

- *Carbohydrate and fat metabolism*

- *Production of hormones in the adrenal gland*

- *Skin and nervous system*

- *Stress resistance*

- *Normal growth of all the cells of the body*

Lack of B5 can lead to:

- *Pain in the nerves, particularly in hands and feet*

- *Headaches*

- *Unusual fatigue*

- *Mental disturbances*

- *Irritability*

- *Defects in the large and small intestine*

B6 (Pyridoksine) Important for:

- *Fat metabolism*

- *Protein metabolism*

- *The creation of red blood cells*

Lack of B6 can lead to:

- *Skin irritations and spots*

- *Eczema and related skin problems*

- *Seborrhoea*

- *Anaemia*

- *Cramps*

- *Morning sickness during pregnancy*

- *Nervousness/ mental problems*

- *Dyspepsia*

- *Cavities (more than normal)*

- *Bloated face*

B12 (Colbalamine) Important for:

- *Enzymatic systems and the distribution of amino acids*

- *Protein metabolism*

- *Fat and sugar metabolism*

- *The central nervous system*

- *Skin and other tissues*

- *Antibodies*

Lack of B12 can lead to:

- *Anaemia*

- *Sore mouth and tongue*

- *Stiffness and pain in the back*

- *Problems with menstruation*

- *Changes in the central nervous system*

Folic Acid Important for:

- *Without enough folic acid, the cells cannot duplicate and grow*

- *It's vital for all normal processes of life*

- *Maturing of red blood cells*

- *Manufacturing of anti-bodies*

- *The cell division*

Lack of Folic Acid can lead to:

- *Anaemia*

- *Fatigue*

- *Pale skin*

- *Dizziness*

- *Depression*

- *Greyish-brown pigmentation spots*

PABA (Para amino benzoic acid) Important for:

- *The assimilation and use of proteins, fats, and carbohydrates*

- *Growth factor for several micro organisms*

- *Protects against sunburn and premature ageing of skin and tissues*

Lack of PABA can lead to:

- *Not well known, but it's assumed it can lead to anaemia, pigment spots and fatigue*

Inositol Important for:

- *Supplement is recommended if you are on a diet or not eating nutritious food*

- *Fat metabolism*

- *Regulating cholesterol levels*

Lack of Inositol can lead to:

- *Obstipation*

- *Elevated cholesterol levels*

- *Eczema and skin problems*

- *Hair loss*

Biotin

- *A lot is available in normal foods, but if you are on a diet - or eating mainly fast foods and processed food, you should be careful.*

Important for:

- *The normal functions of your skin*

Lack of Biotin can lead to:

- *Flaky, dry, and irritated skin*

- *Muscle pains*

- *Loss of appetite*

- *Depression*

- *Fatigue*

- *Loss of hair*

- *Respiratory infections*

Summary

As you probably have noticed, all the B vitamins play important parts in your nervous system, as well as in the health, look, and normal functions of your skin and hair. Deficiencies show very quickly on your outside, with skin problems that cannot be fixed by medicines, serums, or creams. Skin cells must be fed the right food for health. It takes three weeks for new cells to show on the surface, so supplements need this time to work.

The B Complex is absolutely the key to solving a lot of problems with the nervous system, from depression to general lack of energy and zest for life. It's easy and absolutely risk free to start taking complete supplements, and you can add Brewer's Yeast and Pollen for a super energy boost for the body and soul.

Stress and water-soluble vitamins

I will start with the lifestyle factors that deplete your body of whatever B vitamins it has. Stress is the number one culprit, and number two is sugar. Stress burns off vitamin Bs, and to metabolize sugar and sweets, the B team needs to be constantly restocked. What happens if you do not refill your depleted storage? You will get all kinds of visible skin problems, allergies, and immune problems.

A lack of B complex will make you nervous and depressed

You will gradually become nervous, depressed and unfocused, with a lack of energy and totally out of sync with life. Your hair will look lifeless and your skin will look dehydrated and blotchy. The good news is that everybody who has slipped into this black hole of reality can get back their zest for living as well as a healthy, glossy exterior by something so simple as taking B complex supplements.

Nervous breakdown due to lack of B complex

I will share a story with you that really opened my eyes to the severe consequences of vitamin B deficiency. In the eighties, I had made the first formula for a complete vitamin-mineral supplement in Norway: VitaMineral Plus.

I was cooperating closely with the research department of one of the leading pharmaceutical companies in the field, the head professor was a particularly intelligent guy with lots of knowledge.

I was an autodidact in nutrition and biochemistry, but I also possessed the ability to collect, organize and create new solutions that the experts had not even considered.

Then his sister, married to a well-known (and rather pompous) physician, gave birth and immediately went into a post-natal depression and nothing traditional medicine had to offer worked. After I discussed the importance of the B complex with the professor, he obtained pure liquid B complex and gave his sister an injection as this is the fastest route to see an effect. She immediately started to refocus and embraced her newborn baby with joy. Many of the medical team had to admit to the power of vitamins over modern medicine.

Chapter 22

MINERALS ARE OUR LINK TO THE EARTH

Minerals are actually our connection with the earth, the stones, the ocean and the elements. It's rather ingenious that we can get the elements from the soil, clay, and stones into our bodies from the natural world that surrounds us. It shows how we really are a part of the whole universe, and that the balance of it all affects every one of us.

The Macro Minerals

Sodium (salt, Na)

Your body contains approximately 90 grams (in your bones), so salt is important for osmotic pressure, which is the regulation of the body's water balance. Normally, food provides sufficient amounts, so beware of using extra as it can cause high blood pressure. Too much can also have a negative effect on your kidneys. If you are in the tropics and sweat a lot, you might need supplements. Heavy diarrhoea also requires extra salt and plenty of water.

Potassium

Your body contains around 140 grams, 90% of which is stored in your cells. It's the most important cation in extracellular fluid. Eat enough vegetables like cucumber, tomatoes, carrots and fruit juices to cover your needs. Bananas are also an excellent source.

Calcium and Phosphor

Your body contains approx. 1.2 kg calcium and 2 kg phosphor. Your bones and teeth consist of 60 to 70% calcium and phosphor. Calcium is needed for the membranes of your cells, the function of your heart muscle, the contractions of skeletal muscles, and has the ability to regulate nerve cells and coagulate blood. The relation between calcium and phosphorus will probably influence absorption.

Vitamin D is required to absorb these minerals. Food with a satisfactory level of calcium will normally cover your need for phosphor too.

Magnesium

This mineral is stored selectively in cells and bones. Magnesium and potassium are dominating cations in all living cells, and they are normally tied to proteins. Magnesium is very important for enzymatic processes and for maintaining the electric potential in nerves and muscle membranes.

A depletion of magnesium can lead to arrhythmia (irregular heartbeats), as well as cramps and mental disturbances.

Trace minerals Iron

Iron is very important for your blood and different enzymatic systems in your body. A lack of iron can gradually lead to anaemia, and you will be pale, feel exhausted, suffer headaches, dizziness etc. It's also important for the menstrual cycle. The absorption of iron requires enough Vitamin C and Vitamin E.

Copper

This mineral is stored in your tissues and kidneys. It's important in certain enzymatic processes, including iron utilization. If you lack copper, your immune system will malfunction. Foods provide 2 to 5 mg, but the FDA recommended intake is 7 mg. Don't overdose, as intake over 10 mg can lead to vomiting and diarrhoea.

Zinc

Zinc is important in many enzymatic processes. It's stored in small quantities, and you can easily be deficient if you don't get enough in your daily foods. A lack of zinc means your immune defense will be weakened, you will lose your appetite, and experience skin problems. Cuts, bruises and sores will not heal properly either. There may also be stunted growth and generally reduced cell activity.

Zinc is a catalyst for the absorption of the other minerals, so a lack of zinc can lead to dangerous deficiencies. The recommended daily allowance is 15 mg for adults.

Manganese

Deficiencies have not been observed in humans, as it's abundant in basic foods like eggs, grains, whole wheat our and brown bread, beans, nuts, and yeast.

Iodine

This is an essential mineral for the adequate production of the hormones, thyroxine and trijodotyronin, both important for normal metabolism. The thyroid gland contains normally 8 to 10 mg iodine, which is 70 to 80% of the total amount stored in the body.

If you lack thyroxine, more or less all the mental and physical processes in the body are inhibited and lowered. Low levels will also lead to weight gain, increased fat storage, and a lack of energy.

Excess levels lead to goitre and struma (when the thyroid gland increases in size and your eyes protrude visibly). Operation is necessary, and a daily supplement of thyroxin is a must. The most important sources of this vital mineral are shellfish, kelp, and algae. If you don´t eat fish or seafood at least a couple of times a week, you are at risk, so take supplements.

Fluoride

This mineral is stored in your bones and teeth. It's a caries inhibitor, and it's also used together with calcium to battle osteoporosis. It's added to toothpaste to protect the teeth, but this is a matter of debate. Fluoride exists naturally in soil but varies enormously from district to district.

Molybden

Deficiencies have not been observed, as the daily allowance is easy to obtain from meat, grains, beans, lentils, etc.

Chromium

This mineral is crucial for the normal metabolism of sugar and starches and for regulation of the blood sugar levels. If you don´t have enough, you can easily have issues with insulin production. It's vital for the glucose metabolism, and it's possibly a co-factor with insulin to produce satisfactory levels of the glucose tolerance factor necessary for regulating blood sugar levels in order for insulin to work.

Chromium is also of important for the cardiovascular system and for maintaining normal levels of fat in the blood.

It you lack chromium, you will crave sugar, sweets, biscuits and other carbs. Supplements can help a lot to reduce these dangerous cravings. Chromium is found in whole grains, yeast, meat and cheese.

Selenium

This is a vital antioxidant protecting your cells from attack and damage by free oxygen radicals. Selenium is also important for protecting the heart and circulatory system. It's recommended in very high doses following the removal of amalgam fillings (both for the dentist and the patient) to avoid health problems. Natural food sources are kidneys, liver, and seafood.

Chapter 23

POLLUTION AND NEED FOR NUTRIENTS

We have to realise that all the man-made components that we are exposed to each day have side effects that we know little about. How does it influence our mental and physical health? How does it influence our absorption of nutrients?

When you do some research and ask difficult questions, you often end up with even bigger questions. As a journalist and chief editor of Shape-Up Magazine, I have been doing in-depth research that has found some worrying results.

Medicines are mega business
- with serious side effects

The lack of long-term consequence thinking, hunting for patients as regular consumers, is clearly the wrong approach for the future. It may be lucrative in the short term, but it will ultimately lead to the collapse of our healthcare systems.

If we don't start to take responsibility for our own health, we will doom future generations. Those who care about their health and lifestyle will refuse to pay for the consequences of people with damaging lifestyles.

What do you lack?

I listed the most common symptoms of deficiency under the description of different vitamins and minerals to help you recognize the source of any symptoms. It's very common that we need a little extra because of our modern lifestyle and stresses that influence our requirements. As these compounds work together, a lack of one or more can create a domino effect of reactions (or lack of) in your whole body

Your body needs calcium, potassium, phosphorus, iodine, copper, zinc, selenium, etc. They are of vital importance as building materials for your cells to ensure that all metabolic processes will function in a normal, healthy way.

The content of minerals in the body is not constant it will change. For instance, your bones renew every 7 to 10 years, while the bones of children are renewed in just a couple of years.

Industrial foods are depleted

Modern food manufacturing technology, worldwide distribution and long-term storage, combined with the use of a lot of dangerous pesticides and other products to increase production, in influence the mineral balance of the earth as well as the nutritional content of the harvests. Unfortunately, it is difficult to fully comprehend the impact this has.

We do know this influences the content of vitamins and minerals in our food, and it could contribute to the emergence of new health problems as our bodies are unable to adapt to the good of new elements introduced to us. The result is that our health is under serious attack and is being deprived of the necessary nutrition it.

You can protect yourself and your family by taking some basic steps in your daily life. Avoid buying foods with a long shelf life and lots of additives. Avoid foods and drinks that contain empty calories, complex chemical ingredients, and lots of sugar, carbs, fats (particularly trans fats), sweeteners, artificial tastes and colouring.

If you don't understand the names in the ingredients lists, avoid or search the internet for information. Science has proved that a correct balance of nutrients is important for your body and brain.

I think daily supplements are a must today, as we probably need higher doses to combat the challenges of our new world. Of course, supplements should add to varied natural foods and drinks and a healthy lifestyle.

Aqua Vita, Water of Life

When we talk about vital nutrients, it's easy to forget water. Water is a vital nutrient too, and without it, we would die pretty quickly. The other nutrients in our body last longer and are depleted at a far slower rate, but water is needed on a daily basis, so it's actually the most important of all nutrients.

Water is a must for the metabolic processes of all your cells. It's crucial for the transport of oxygen, nutrients and toxins in the intracellular fluids, the gut, and its surroundings.

Water is also a cooler, and it's very important to keep shape and form of the cells and soft tissues. Enough water each day is necessary for skin health too and it's definitely nature's very best moisturizer. Just visualize a tempting, juicy apricot and a dried one, to a plump, mouthwatering grape and a wrinkly raisin. The difference between hydrated and dehydrated is the same in human skin.

You are a water baby

50 to 75 % of your body weight is water. All of us need at least 1,100 ml each day, in addition to the 500 to 900 ml of water we get in our foods. In addition, around 400 ml is produced in your body. It evaporates via:

- *Skin and lungs: 900 – 1,000 ml*

- *Faeces: 80 – 100 ml*

- *Urine: 1,000 – 1,300 ml*

Beware of dehydration

A loss of 5% of body weight leads to a loss of energy and reduced ability to function. A loss of 12% is very dangerous and can cause death. Transpiration of more than 5 to 10% means a high risk for lack of salt, which could induce cramps. Lots of water is a must if you have diarrhoea, and for children it's vital for survival!

Stress, alcohol, coffee, heat, transpiration, anxiety, fever and diarrhoea are among the factors that contribute to dehydration. So, beware and drink enough during the day to keep your body and mind functioning smoothly.

The older we get, the less thirst we feel, so it's easy to forget. Do you crave to eat? Sometimes we misjudge the signals from our brain to our bodies and the body needs to be filled up with water, not food. Just try it. Instead of reaching for a snack, drink some water.

Plastic – not fantastic

Avoid drinking from plastic bottles, as the chemicals in the plastic are not good for you. In addition, these water bottles are contributing to the pollution and the contamination as well as ruin of our oceans and nature.

Buy a good non-toxic metal bottle for carrying around and use only glass bottles at home. Keep a bottle in your living room, the kitchen, your bedroom and your home office so you can remember to drink regularly.

Chapter 24

SPEED UP YOUR LIFE AND START MOVING

Your new firm and fit body

The great challenge on the road to rejuvenation is quite simply exercise. Even if fitness is a big business and lots of people work out on a daily basis, many of us just don´t. We have millions of excuses for postponing our good intentions to tomorrow or next week.

Many are afraid of leaving their comfort zone. It's "I know what I have but I don´t know what I get". Many think it's better to stay put and avoid risks.

The excuses for a sedentary life are varied, but this unfortunately has the same negative effects for us as they are stopping us from using our bodies in the way we should.

We are constructed for movement if we want all the complex processes of our organs, cells, hormones, neurotransmitters, immune system etc. to work normally. Our body will literally rust and gradually malfunction if it's not used.

Sedentary lifestyle has a high price

A lot of women have a low metabolism due to a lack of activity combined with a body composition high in fatty tissue and low in lean muscle mass. Muscles require energy to work, and they burn calories, but fat deposits are passive storage space. Dieting has also made a lot of women fat! Each time we lose weight without training to maintain muscle mass, we lose muscle mass as well as fat.

The result is a lower resting metabolism – meaning that you need a lower food intake to avoid putting on more weight.

Each diet without training leaves us fatter than before and ruins our metabolism. We can "eat like a bird" but still be fat. It's a sad fact that many women end up on a lifelong yo-yo regime of weight loss – increase – diet – weight loss – increase... What started as a small problem can end up a very, very big one.

Reverse – increase – and normalize

The key to a normal metabolism is movement and developing more muscle. That means some exercise every day. In this book, find some of my favourite exercises from my Slim Trim regime. It's easy to follow, and it gives brilliant results if you just do it.

Thousands of women have followed it, at home as well as in groups and I can tell you the transformations of body and mind have been fantastic.

So, please do yourself an enormous favour: get moving and get your wonderful, healthy body back! You can do it in just 15 to 30 minutes a day in addition to some extra brisk walking and being more focused on staying on your legs more often than on your bum.

You will burn more fat

The good news is that when you alter the ratio between muscles and fat, your metabolism will increase –24/7. You will get fitter and leaner, and you will have loads more of energy and a renewed zest for life.

Fat has more volume than muscle

1 kg of muscle requires far less space than 1 kg of fat (have a look the next time you are at the butchers). This means that by altering the fat/ muscle ratio, you can reduce your size and measurements without losing your weight. So, perhaps you will find out that you are not really overweight at all!

Shape up!

You will find the answer when you have measured and weighed yourself and filled in your personal chart. Perhaps you just have too much fat and too little muscle! The great thing is that you can gradually transform the ratio and firm and reshape your body by following the easy routines in my Slim Trim system.

With these super shaping exercises, you will gain muscle mass, and reduce unsightly ab and unwanted fatty deposits. I promise you that you will get you fabulous results quickly. So, just go for it and invest 30 minutes a day in your own looks and wellness. It will be the best investment of your life.

Calculate your ideal weight

Here's a simple way to do it. Take your height in centimetres and subtract 100 cm, which gives you maximum weight (kg) for your height. If you are 160 cm tall, 60 kgs is your maximum weight. Above that means too much in fat deposits, and you need to lose it.

Most women look best if they are 5 to 10 % less, meaning: 54 to 57 kg for a 160 cm tall woman with a normal fat to muscle ratio.

Measure your waist

The dangerous fat deposits are around your waist and stomach. If you are a woman with a measurement of 80 cm or more, you are actually in the risk zone for diabetes, heart problems, and other illnesses.

You can have a perfectly normal weight (even be underweight) and still have a dangerous distribution of fat. That is what you have to alter by getting more physical on a daily basis.

I know from my own experience how tough it is to reduce the middle, as it's also a female hormonal problem after menopause. But we all have to try, because the alternative is far worse than doing some daily exercises and eating healthier.

One on – one off

If you don't need to lose weight but want to get healthier, try the combination of a day or two on the Detox Diet per week, combined with the Slim Trim regime. I promise it will give you results you can be proud of.

I just do what I have to do....

By the way, if you think I am a fitness freak and LOVE to exercise, you are totally wrong. I do it because I have to if I want to keep my looks, my figure, my health and actually look and feel younger than my actual age. It's an investment in myself, even if I love to relax with my feet up reading a good book.

I get up because I do NOT want to look like me a little old lady. I was born in 1941 and I am still alive and kicking. I feel like my normal grown up self, not a wobbly senior citizen. I am lucky with my health, my body and my looks, but I need maintenance and care, and it costs nothing but a little daily effort.

Your body – vintage and valuable – or straight to the heap?

My dear friend, you are the owner of the most precious vehicle ever in your life: Your body!! Pamper, polish and use it and keep it running smoothly on the right kind of fuel. It can survive almost anything if looked after, and movement is the number one thing to keep the engine running!

My Slim Trim program is based on yoga

I love yoga, as these ancient – yet modern – exercises are so extremely effective for health and fitness. They are really (in my opinion) superior because they improve your total body. It reduces stress and works for your brain and your soul too. It's a very scientific system of total fitness and wellbeing that can rejuvenate and restore you from inside out.

No matter what age, shape and size, you can find yoga positions that are suitable for you to gradually become stronger, more flexible and downright healthier. Do not let the weird names of the exercises turn you off even if they sound rather foreign and far out.

It's just because most are from ancient Indian Sanskrit, and they are actually describing what the exercises look like, which makes them easier to remember.

Yoga is the core of fitness

Most fitness programs I have created are based on yoga exercises, but to make them more suited to modern women, I combine them with static, strengthening exercises and maximized the cardiovascular effect by using Western music. It gives more energy than the relaxing Indian music that can sound foreign to our ears.

Evas Shape-Up System

I used what I believed in and what I knew was working! I named my fitness system Shape-Up. It worked like a charm, and nobody suspected that ancient Indian yoga was the source of this very cool, disco fitness system. I trained hundreds of Eva Shape-Up instructors all over the country. Local classes (as well as personal training and nutrition/ diet advice) got thousands and thousands of women out of their comfy couches!

Start NOW. This will melt your love handles. This will flatten your muffin top. The messages and motivations and the exercises are still the same! Why?? Because they work, they are fun, and they give visible results mega-fast!

Set your limits

I think your body sets limits by sending pain signals. So, when you do exercise, move until you reach your limit and then push a little more. Increase gradually as you get stronger, leaner, fitter and more flexible.

Take time to focus on your muscles focus on how your body works and visualize your muscles getting firmer, stronger and younger again - and gradually you will turn it into reality. Respect your body and care for it with enough movement to make it work properly throughout your whole life.

Remember, you are made for movement not for sitting. If you don't use your body or challenge it, it will gradually deteriorate.

My motto is: Lots of gain and no pain

Take care of your wonderful body and maintain it with daily exercises. Even small doses are far better than none. I hope I can remove all excuses and obstacles and make it really easy and fun for you to firm up and strengthen your body without a lot of effort and planning. Just make it part of the way you use your body in your daily life. I can promise you these exercises are life and looks savers, and rejuvenators for body and soul! This is one of the most important secrets of good health and a rm and t body no matter what age you are. So, get cracking for your own sake!!

Enjoy the results!

Chapter 25

YOUR DAILY FITNESS PROGRAM

I have put together my favourites in a daily dozen that are extremely easy to do without any equipment other than your own body. You can actually do many of them anywhere at your own leisure, no matter what level of fitness you start from. Some of them you can even do sitting down until you get stronger. First of all, you should learn to breathe efficiently, as enough oxygen is the key to a healthy body and mind.

Stress is dangerous, and fattening

Sometimes it seems impossible to reduce weight (or avoid putting it on). You feel you eat like a bird, but the pounds keep piling on! You feel fat and depressed when you try on clothes. Your self-confidence is low, and your stress levels are elevated to new heights.

Reduce stress, lose weight

The reason for your problem can be stress and a hormonal imbalance. Stress releases cortisol, a hormone that increases the fat storage ability of the body. The excess fat will mainly be deposited around the middle part of the body, so you lose your waistline and get the middle-aged pot belly.

You must relax to lose weight

Stress management and relaxation are important for anybody wanting to reduce their weight and measurements.

That is why you need to look at your total lifestyle to reduce the stress and learn techniques to handle it. Some mental training and motivation forms part of this book. It's important that you master your mind as well as your body, as they must be in balance for you to feel well and happy in your body and soul. The key to reducing stress is to learn breathing techniques. They are also important for your fitness level and general health, so start now and use them on a daily basis. It does take a little time and patience in the start, but it will certainly do you a world of good!

Basic Breathing Techniques

You need enough oxygen for efficient metabolism. To increase your level, you should start your day – your fitness program – with the simple breathing exercises based on yoga. I can assure you that they work, and that you will feel fitter, have better skin, and release stress and related problems.

Blow on the fire

Sit relaxed on the floor in a yoga position with your legs crossed under you. Straighten your back, lower your shoulders and stretch your neck. Look straight ahead. Start by breathing in through your nose and fill your lungs as much as possible. Hold for a second, then slowly, slowly release the air through pursed lips (like blowing out a candle). Empty the lungs completely so you have to draw in air through your nose.

Fill yourself all the way down to the stomach. The deeper the better. Hold, and release slowly. Repeat as many times as you can. Focus on your breathing and visualize your breaths as waves on the seashore: the regular, strong, in and out of the ocean to the shore. It can help to visualize it. You can also use music with ocean sounds.

This can help to erase stress and help you to stay in the now, increasing your mindfulness.

Airing and strengthening your lungs

Many of us just breath with the upper part of the chest. When we tuck our tummies in, our breathing gets superficial. Stale air is collected, and your lungs (and your complete airway system) need a good "clean out". It's easier than you think, and it will give you amazing results if you do this on a daily basis.

Deep breathing will stress you down

I am talking from experience, as this helped me to combat serious stress problems that gave me heart problems some years ago. Breathing and yoga (combined with cleaning up feelings and personal relationships) was far better than the medicine and surgery the doctors recommended.

Of course, you should always listen to your doctors and their advice, but you should also do enough research to be able to discuss your health challenges and find a solution that feels right for you.

Be sensible and neutral and show respect for different opinions. It's your body – it's your life. So, start up with getting enough of the essence of life: oxygen.! Learn how to breath, relax and enjoy.

Sit relaxed in the yoga position

Rest your hands on your knees with your palms facing upwards. Close your eyes so you can focus on your inner self. Start by inhaling as much air as you possibly can through your nose. Fill up so your chest and let your ribcage and stomach expand as much as possible. Then exhale as slowly as possible.

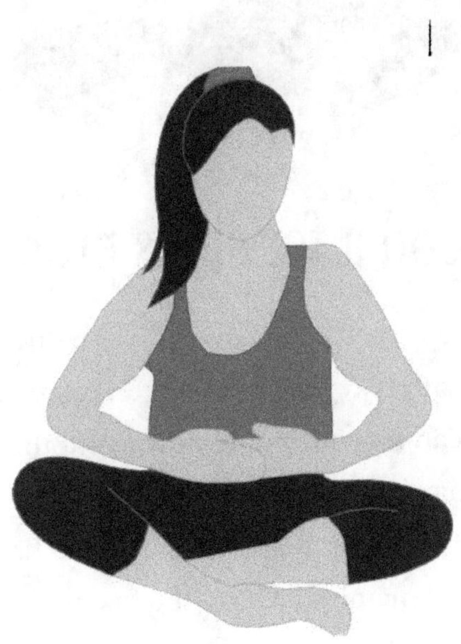

Airing your nostrils

You can gradually add this nostril breathing. Use your index finger to close one nostril. Breath in deeply through the other one. Then switch fingers and close the other nostril and breath out. Repeat until you feel your breathing is easier and deeper and tension is released.

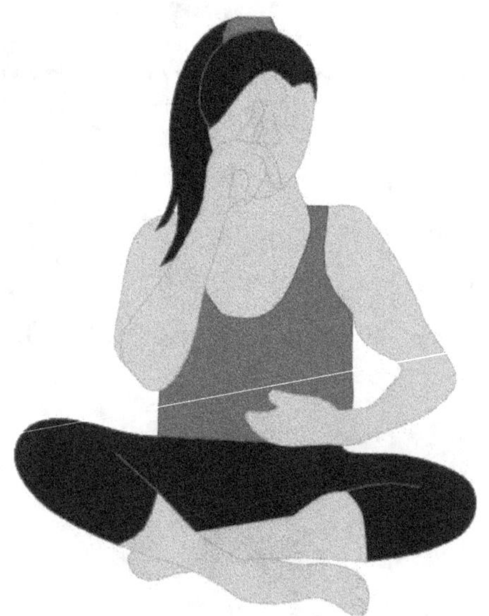

Good a for sinus problems

If you have problems getting enough oxygen due to a clogged nose, it will help to rinse it with lukewarm salt water every morning. Try to sniff up the water so you can feel it running down your throat. In the beginning you must repeat it many times, but gradually it will clear up. When you feel less congested, blow your nose and sniff up a little olive oil to soften and nourish the mucus membranes so they function better.

This is a very good natural cure for sinus trouble too!! Many medical specialists recommend it when medicines don´t work (or to avoid antibiotics).

When you learn these simple breathing techniques, make them part of your daily life. Whenever you feel stressed and you are losing your ability to concentrate, take a few minutes.

You can sit anywhere and in any way you like as long as you lower your shoulders, straighten your back, close your eyes, and start breathing deeply and regularly in through your nose and out of your mouth.

If you are in a situation that makes it difficult, take five and go to the loo. If you are on the tube, train, bus etc., you have a splendid chance to relax with your deep breathing and return home feeling renewed and invigorated.

Chapter 26

EVAS SLIMTRIM

These are super easy exercises that you can do on your living room floor or bedroom. You can master them even if you feel fat, clumsy, and in rotten shape. The reward is that you gradually will feel (and look) firmer, slimmer, more flexible, and stronger.

In a week or two you will find it so easy. Your self-confidence will increase each day you follow the program. As an extra reward from your body-brain, you will increase your resting metabolism by 15% when you exercise for 30 minutes. It will stay higher for the next 12 hours.

You can make an extra effort for yourself and keep it higher for 24 hours with 30 minutes is Slim Trim morning and night. Imagine how many extra fat reserves you will burn off!

If you want a tougher and more challenging program, there are great free fitness videos on YouTube. It doesn't matter what you do. As long as it makes you sweat, you are on the right track to a New You and a new fabulous lifestyle.

Warm up

If you like to dance, why don't you? It's a great way to warm up and get ready for the rest of the exercises. Put on your favourite happy music and go for the ones that you connect with fun and good times. I have lots of old disco music that gets me in the mood and I just love it when I get going! You can also switch to Latino music if you like to move your body in a more sensual way, or you can mix whatever makes you happy.

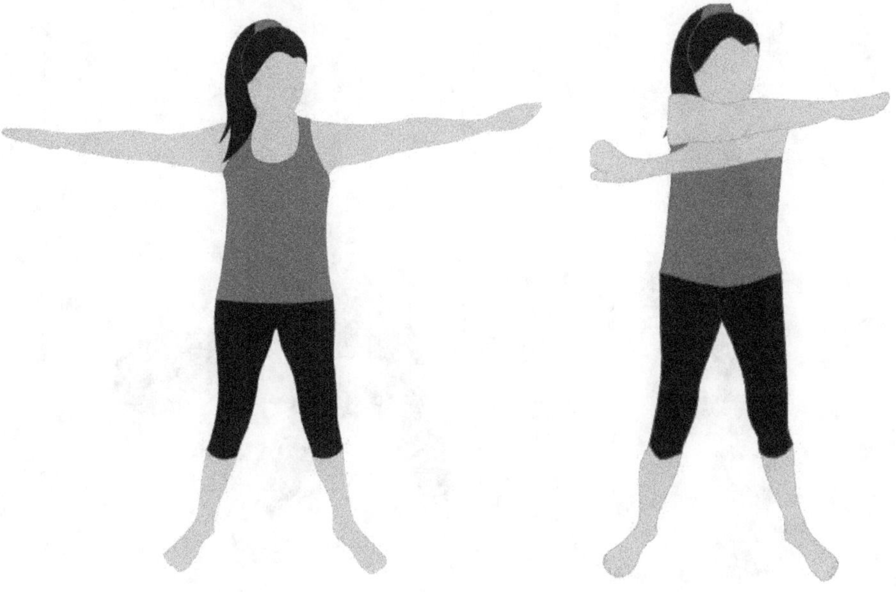

Let your hair out and do exactly what you feel like. Give all you have, feel like a woman, and wriggle and move all you've got. Close your eyes and feel like a goddess.

Remember to breathe – in and out, out and in, from the stomach. Lift your arms, bend down and skip and jump. Do whatever you can to get hot.

An alternative warm up is to use a skipping rope or just walk up and down your living room (and stairs if you have them). As long as you get your heart rate up and breathe harder you are on your way. Do this for a minimum of 10 minutes to kick start your metabolism and burn fat.

You can add these two exercises to your warmup when you are fitter. When you do the crisscross touch your toes exercise, you can bend your knees for extra protection of your back. Just listen to your body – it always knows best!

The jump and touch exercise can be done fast or slow, depending on your fitness level. Lift your left leg and touch the knee with your right elbow, then lift your right knee and touch with left elbow. Alternate, and remember to keep your back straight and your core muscles tight.

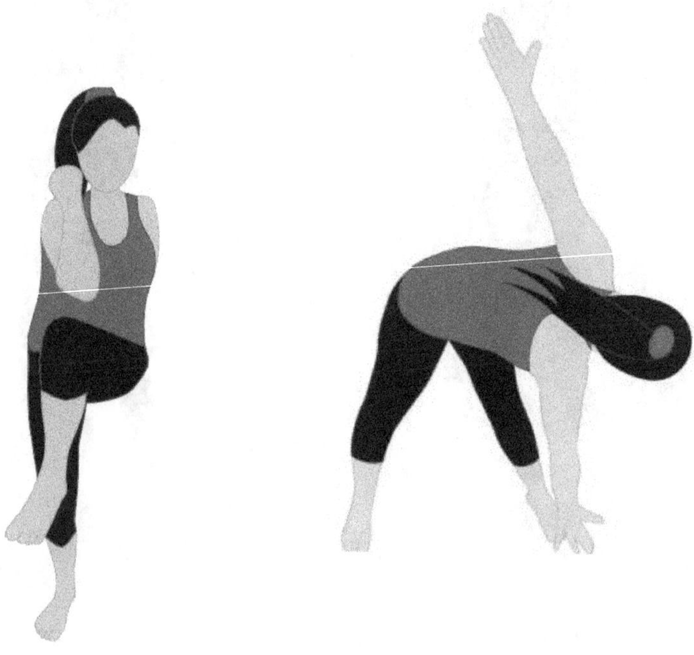

Sit ups for a flatter tummy

Lie down on your yoga mat and press the small of your back toward the floor. Bend your knees and press the soles of your feet into the floor with toes pointing forward. Stretch your back and neck in a straight line.

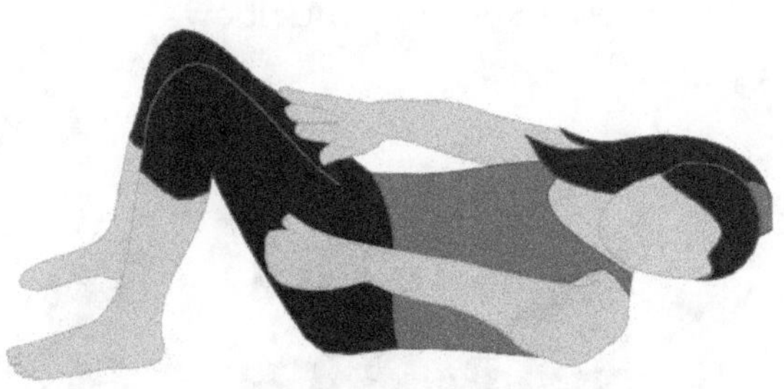

Lift your torso up by using your stomach muscles. Don't bend your neck backwards but keep it in line with your spine. Gradually bend your neck forward and look at your navel. Keep your arms straight out in front of you. Hold the position and count to ten. Relax and repeat 10 times.

Then stretch your arms to the right and repeat 10 times. Then to your left in the same way, 10 repetitions. Feel how the different stomach muscles are working.

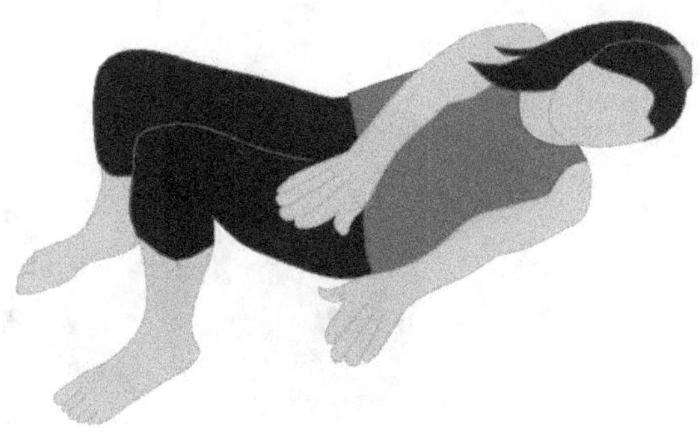

Extra tummy tighteners

When you are lying on your back, you can add these two exercises that are a bit tougher.

Lift your shoulders but keep the small of your back glued to the floor. Look at your navel Lift and bend your right knee and touch your left elbow – and then your left knee to your elbow. You can do it fast or slow, whatever suits you.

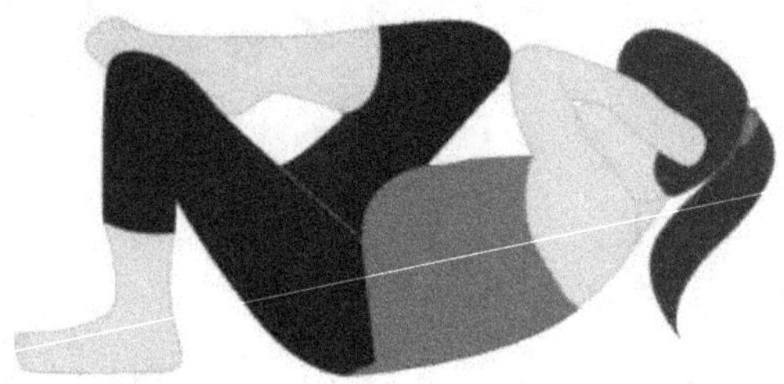

Then you can do make-believe biking. Use your legs forwards, backwards and to the side. Feel the tightening of your stomach muscles! Feel how it gets tougher when you move your legs closer to the floor. You must keep your back to the floor the whole time to protect your spine.

The faster you bike, the more you increase your circulation, so it is a great way to improve you fitness level.

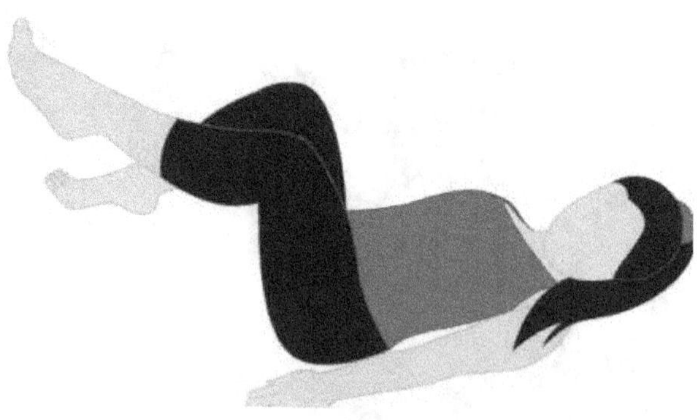

Firmer thighs

Lie on your side (straight line from toes to head). Lean on your elbow and lift your upper leg with a straight knee and pointed toes up and down. Squeeze the muscles of your buttocks. You don't have to lift more than a 60-degree angle. Turn over and repeat with the other leg.

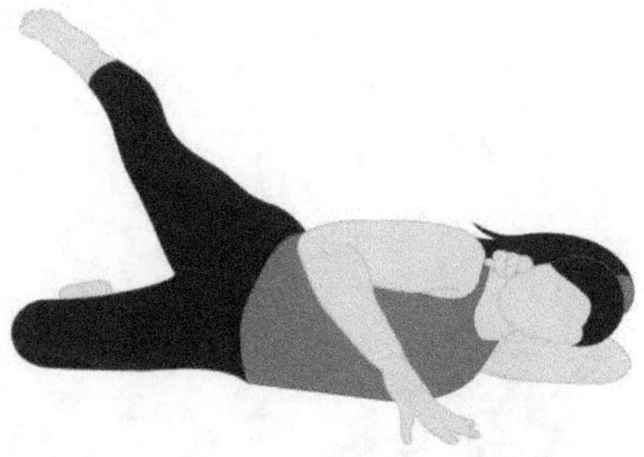

The idea is to build strength and firm up, so try to feel and concentrate on what is happening in your body. Remember to use your core muscles all the time and pull your stomach in. This will help flatten it. Repeat until you give up (at least 20 reps). Count how many you manage and see how rapidly it increases day by day.

Lie in the same position and move your upper leg with a straight knee backwards as far as you can, and then forwards. Repeat 20 times. Turn over and repeat with the other leg.

The next step is to firm up the inner thigh (a weak part for a lot of women). Lie in the same position at on the floor with the lower leg straight and cross the upper leg over your knee with the foot placed at on the floor. Then lift the lower leg up and down and repeat it as many times as possible. You don't have to lift it high, but you must feel that it's really working. Repeat with the other leg.

Extra all over firming

Lie on your back with your arms stretched out to the side, palms down. Press your back to the floor, lift your legs using your core muscles. Feel how they tighten. Then you criss-cross your legs quickly as many repetitions as you can manage. When you are stronger, you can gradually lower your legs during the criss-cross. The lower they are, the tougher the exercise.

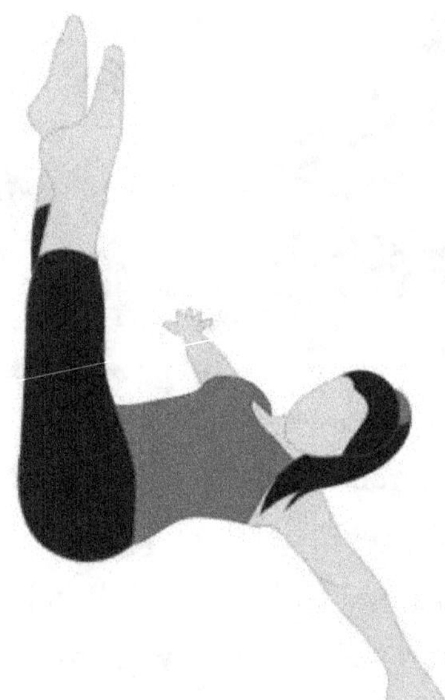

Firmer butt and less cellulite

Start by sitting on the floor in yoga position. Start rolling from side to side so you feel your butt and thighs are getting a hard-kneading massage. If it's difficult to stay balanced, so support yourself by stretching out your arms and steadying yourself with your hands.

Stretch your legs and point your toes and "walk" across the floor using your butt muscles. "Walk" forwards and backwards as much as possible.

Strong and straight

Kneel on all fours. Keep your spine straight! Tuck your tummy towards your spine to protect it. Look straight ahead and stretch out your right arm and leg as far as they can go. Do a minimum of ten repetitions and then repeat with your left side.

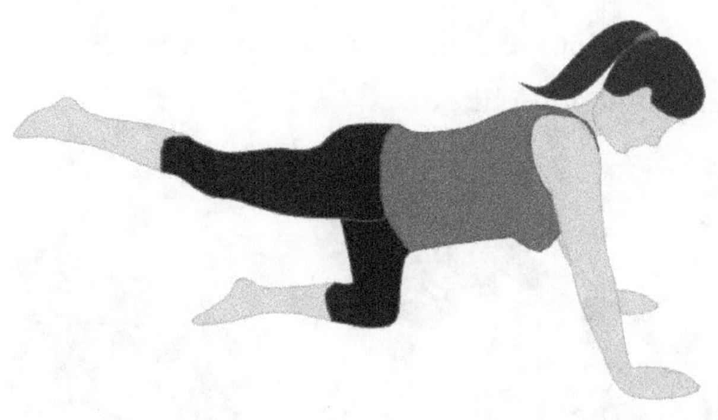

You can also do an easier version if you have problems with your balance on all fours. Lie down on your stomach. Stretch and lift your left arm forward as you lift your right leg up. Keep your knee straight. Feel the muscles in your butt and thigh working. Hold and count to twenty. Relax, count twenty – and lift left leg up, stretch right arm forward. Minimum 10 repetitions to each side.

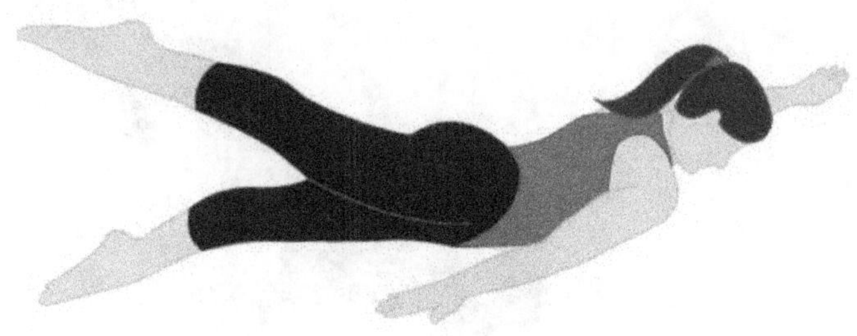

Farewell flip-flop arms

This is a very weak point for women. When we lose muscle tone, the inside of the upper arms starts to sag. Strengthen the muscles to firm up and avoid further sagging. This push-up and stretch exercise combines strengthening your back, butt, thighs as well as your arms.

Stand on all fours, palms pointing forwards, straight elbows. Tighten your tummy to protect the small of your back. Move your back upwards and downwards smoothly like a cat.

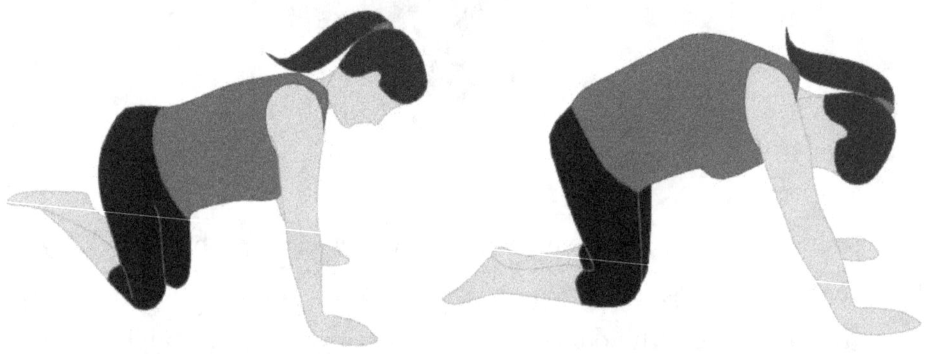

Kneel on your knees, have straight arms with palms on the floor, fingers pointing forwards. Rest on both legs. Bend your elbows and get as near to the floor as possible, keeping a straight spine by using your tummy muscles. Do as many repetitions as you can, slowly and controlled – up and down.

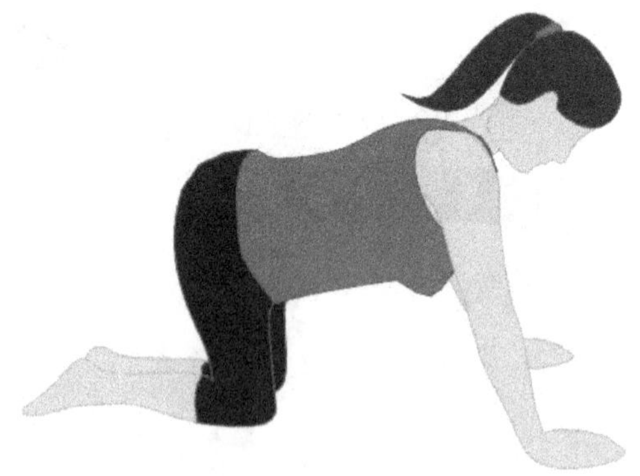

If the push-ups are difficult in the start, you have this is easy and efficient alternative: Stand straight and face towards a wall. Place your palms on the wall with straight arms. Bend the elbows and push against the wall, but keep your back straight. Tighten your muscles as much as you can and then count slowly to 15 and breathe out. Repeat at least ten times. When you are very strong, you can do regular push-ups with straight legs on the floor.

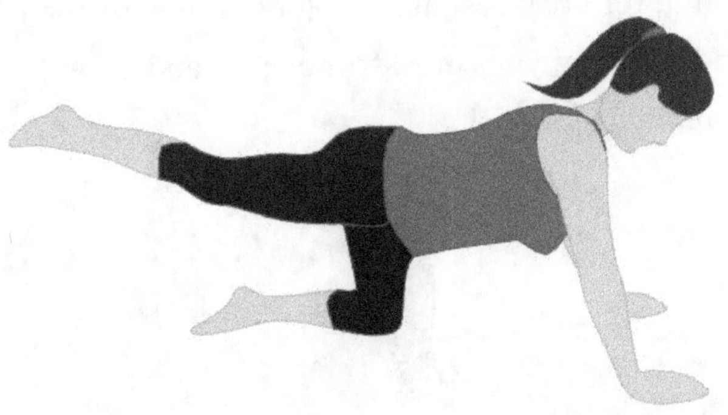

The second part of the exercise is excellent for your back. Stand the same way, and reach out your right arm and your left leg. Stretch out as far as you can. Hold the position as long as possible, then switch to other side. Take as many repetitions as possible. If you have a weak back, I recommend that you this exercise several times a day.

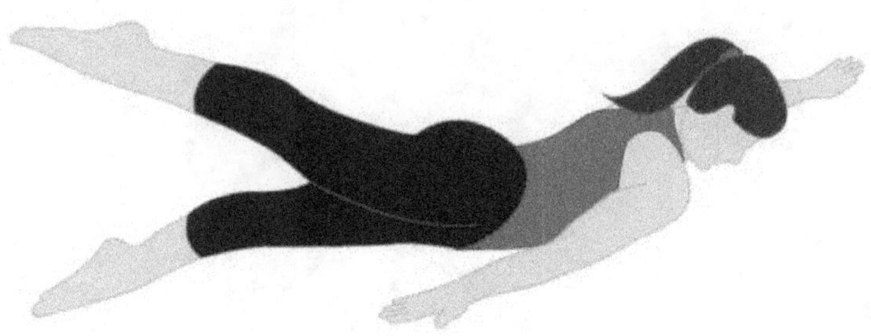

It is even easier if you lie on your stomach and stretch and lift arms and legs, hold and count to ten, relax at ten – and repeat as many times as you can manage.

Tit and Arm lift

This is a static exercise and very efficient and easy to do anywhere. It builds strength in your chest and arm muscles. You can do it sitting or standing. Keep your back straight, with low shoulders and a long neck. Hold your hands (palms) together in front of your chest. Push your hands together as hard as you can and count slowly to 15; relax and repeat as often as possible for great results. Just look in the mirror when you press and relax, and see how your breasts move up and down, which is a sure sign that it's really working!!

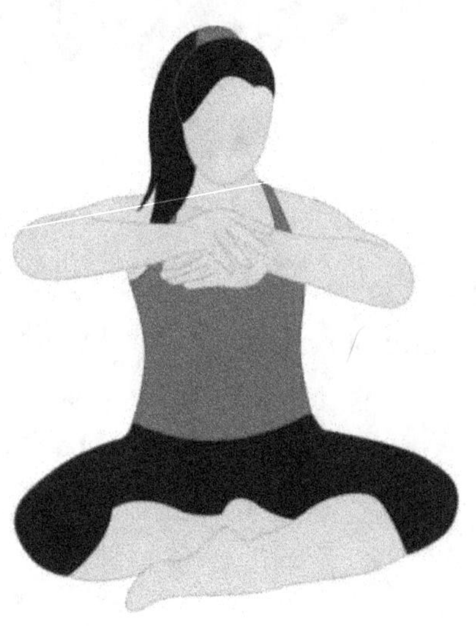

Stretch out and relax

Always finish your fitness session with stretching out. You can start with this ballet inspired stretch. Stand straight, tighten your core and lift your leg up – resting it at table, shelf or chair (depending on your range of motion). Stretch right arm down your right leg and reach as far down as you can while keeping your back as straight as possible. Alternate sides. It is tough to start with, but you will be amazed of your increased flexibility in a very short time. So just do it, every day!

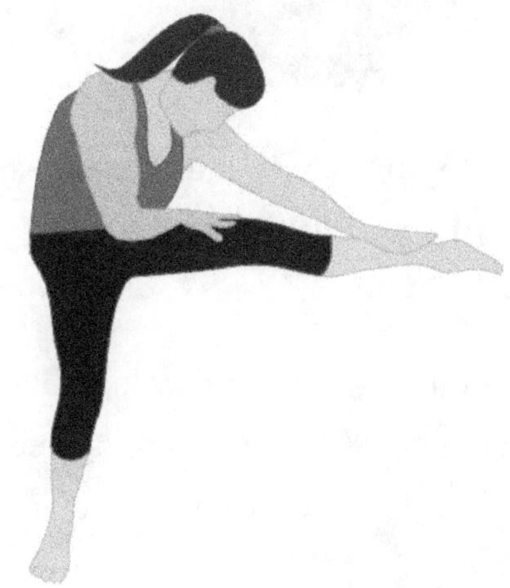

Lie at on your stomach. Bend your knees. Take a firm grip around your legs (as close to your feet as possible) and press towards your butt. Hold, count slowly to fifteen, relax, and repeat at least ten times.

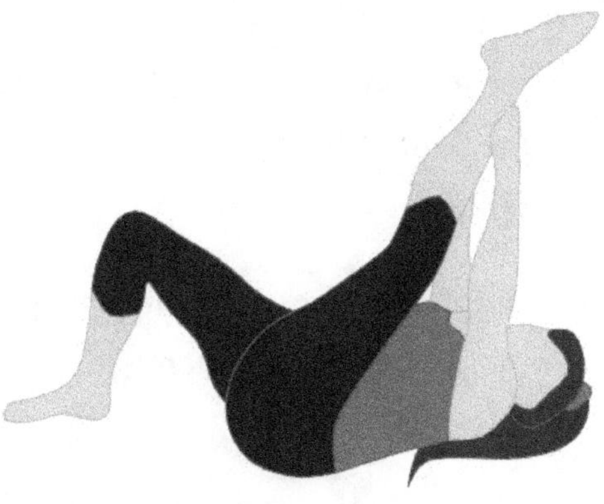

Turn around and lie on your back. Grab your right ankle, keeping your left leg straight, and stretch it toward your chest. Hold, count slowly to fifteen, relax and repeat at least ten times. Remember to keep the small of your back pressed to the floor by using your stomach muscles.

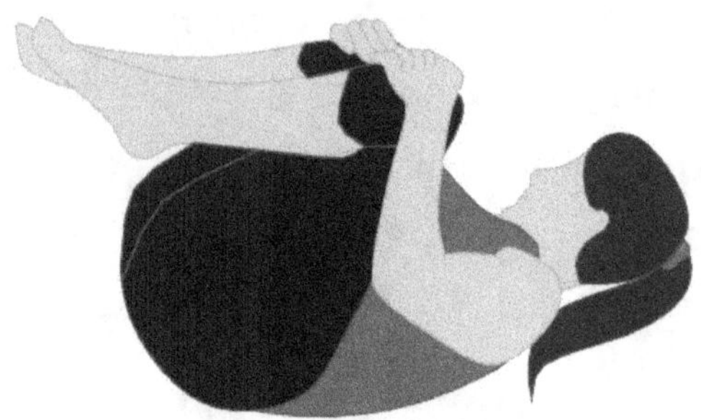

Press your knees to your chest and feel the stretch in buttocks. You can also move on to your stomach, grab your feet and press them towards your butt.

Finish your session lying on your back and place your arms alongside your body, palms facing up. Relax by breathing deeply from your stomach. Feel that your body is getting so heavy and relaxed that you almost sink through the floor.

Do you have problems relaxing?

Lie on your back and breathe deeply. Tighten all your muscles as much as you can. Start with your toes, your legs, your knees, thighs, vagina, butt, back, diaphragm, chest, arms, jaw, and your whole face. Tighten, tighten, tighten until you cannot hold it any longer, then let go and feel what total relaxation is like.

If you are very uptight and stressed, you will probably have to do this exercise several times and repeat it often until you get the hang of it.

But once you learn it, it can be a great help to you. When you really master it, you can do it sitting and standing as well if you need a quick distressing break in your day. This exercise is also brilliant for those who have problems falling asleep. Do it – and at the same time repeat a mantra to relax and "wash" your brain. You can use OHM, the sound of the universe from Ayurvedic medicine. It's extremely calming. Just try, and gradually you will succeed.

Static exercises build muscles

Be more body conscious and learn a few static exercises. You can actually firm up your butt, your thighs, your chest, and your belly when you brush your teeth, relax on a sun bed (or in your bed...), or sit watching your favourite TV program.

The principle is easy: You tighten a muscle group like your stomach muscles and pull them in as hard as you can. Hold the position as long as you can then relax and tighten again.

To learn the technique, stand naked in front of a mirror and see how the muscles move. Tighten, hold and count to at least 15, relax, count to 15 and repeat.

Static mini strengtheners

What about improving your body while you watch your favourite TV program, Netflix or the news? You can even sit in the sofa and do "silent work outs".

What about lifting and tighten up your sagging bum by using your gluteus maximus and pressing them together until your eyes pop, then relax and repeat.

Or perhaps you should firm up your arm muscles by making hard fists and then bending your arms slowly upwards – like lifting weights. Actually, you can fill bottles with water (1 liter) and use them as free weights.

You can also lift your breasts (the underlying chest muscles) by holding your hands together in front of your chest and press hard (see your breasts raise), count to 15 then relax (see them go south).

Get out of the couch during the advertising breaks and make them kick you into firming up your thighs and legs. How? Just stand up straight with your arms stretched out in front of you in shoulder height. Bend your knees, and squat as low as you can. Difficult? Hold on to a chair or a table to start with.

Do the same squat every time you go to the loo, and never ever hold on to sink to get up. Build muscles so you can stay steady and safe on your feet.

To stay fit and as young and strong as possible, it is also important to keep your balance. Daily training does the trick. Stand straight, arms out to the sides in shoulder height. Lift your knee to your chest (pointed toes). Count as far as you can get before you must steady yourself and lower your leg. Switch legs. Do as many repetitions as possible and set yourself goals for how far you can count and still stay steady. Alternate the balance exercise with open and closed yes.

Weak feet and joints are increasing the risk of falling and breaking bones. Stay steady on your feet by doing a simple exercise like standing on flat feet, then lifting your heels and stand on your toes, back – lift again, as many repetitions as you manage.

Pelvic training is vital for you

You can tighten your pelvic floor and keep your vagina fit by remembering to lift the inner pelvic muscles, hold and count to 10, relax and count to 10, and repeat as often as possible.

This can really improve bladder/ anus control and prevent problems as years go by. It's a problem nobody speaks about, but it affects many a woman who has given birth.

As we get older, the connective tissue weakens due to hormonal changes and this results in incontinence and lack of bladder control. The best way to prevent and cure it is to do the pelvic exercises religiously, as often as you remember, but at least morning and evening when you cleanse your skin and brush your teeth.

Why resistance training?

It seems too easy. There's no heavy-duty equipment, actually no equipment besides your own body. Static exercises – resistance training – are proven to build maximum muscle in minimum time.

The Naval Academy in Norway used them as a muscle building supplement when training officer candidates. They called it resistance training and muscle building, and some research showed it was a superior method for achieving rapid and excellent results. My ex-husband was an instructor there, and he was living proof that it worked.

So, use your own body as a resistance tool to build muscle and firm up the ab fast. Do this:

- *In front of the bathroom mirror every morning and evening when you brush your teeth*

- *During TV advertising breaks*

- *When you do the dishes and when you cook*

- *When you are waiting for somebody or something*

- *When you are on public transport*

- *When you have nothing better to do*

I did these tightening exercises every morning for years when I drove from my house in Drammen to Oslo for work. Instead of getting frustrated being stuck in traffic, I put on some great music and tightened, relaxed, tightened. I strengthened my arms, chest and upper back muscles by holding hard on to the steering wheel, contracting on ten, relaxing and repeating.

Sometimes I was stuck like forever, and then I did the same static exercises for my stomach muscles (just pulling them in and counting as far as possible), my butt (tightening gluteus maximus the same way) – my pelvic floor muscles.

Once you get to know your own body and your muscles, it is easy to build any muscles doing static exercises anytime - anywhere.

Chapter 27

YOGA SURYANAMASKAR, SUN SALUT

This is a classic and one of the most well-known yoga exercises. It's done as a continuous movement in 12 steps that oat into each other. It looks more complicated than it is, and the way to learn it properly is to practice each of the steps before you start to do it in one fluid routine. Whatever your shape and form, you can do it. Gradually you will get the hang of it.

Let your body set the limit to the stretches (remember a little is better than nothing). Surprisingly quickly you will see that you get stronger and more flexible. You will have better balance and increase your breathing capacity and your circulation. Gradually you will learn to synchronize your breathing with your movements, and you will feel marvelous as you get better control over your mind and body.

Slow or fast?

You can practice this slowly and stay in the end positions counting to ten before you go on to the next step. This is relaxing and you can meditate while you do it. Or you can do it in a more dynamic way and move quickly and rapidly from one step to another. Let your breathing "drag" you! Repeat several times to get your temperature up and get sweaty. It's good for your body and metabolism.

1. Breathe out

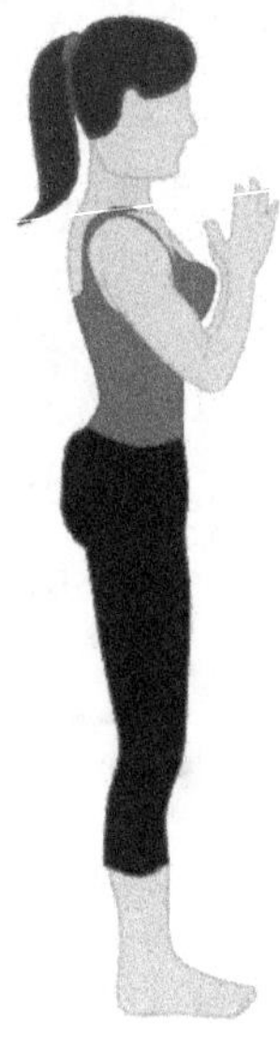

Stand straight with feet together and toes pointing forward. Hold your palms together in front of your chest. Fingers pointing up. Lock your thumbs together.

Stretch upwards and be the tallest version of yourself. Relax your shoulders. Breathe slowly out.

2. . Breathe in

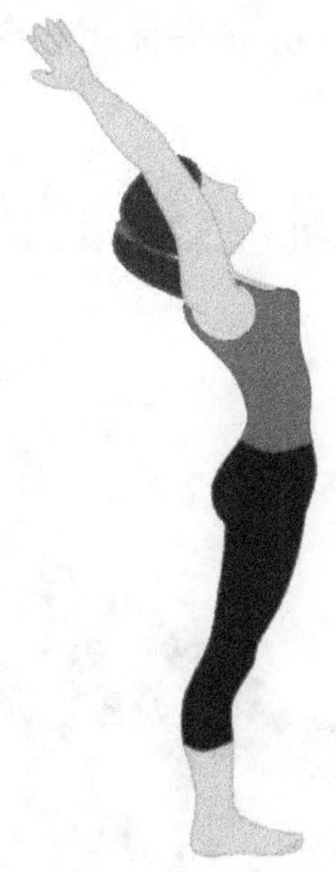

Stretching your arms upwards and backwards. Keep the thumbs locked. Feel that you are bending in the small of your back.

3. Breathe out

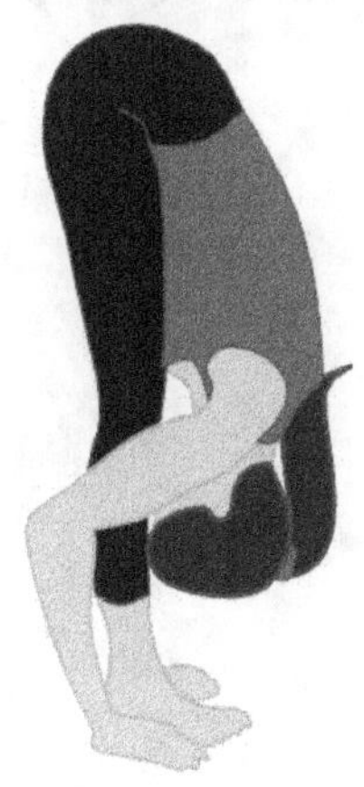

Bend towards the floor. Try to touch the floor with the palms of your hands (on the side of your feet). Keep your knees straight, bend your head as far against your knees as possible and keep your stomach muscles tight all the time. Difficult?

Just go as far as you can in each position and gradually you will be more flexible.

4 . Breathe in

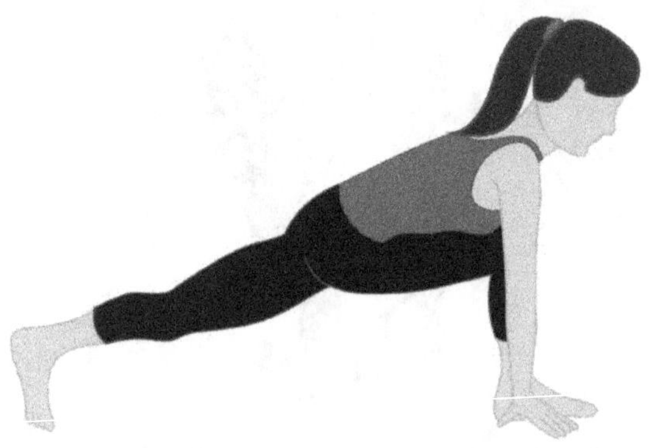

Push your left leg backwards. Your palms (or fingertips) are still touching the floor. Your right knee is bent and pressed forward between your arms. Your left leg is bent towards the floor backwards. It's very important that you are stretching your upper torso and neck and avoid to swaying your back.

5. Breathe out

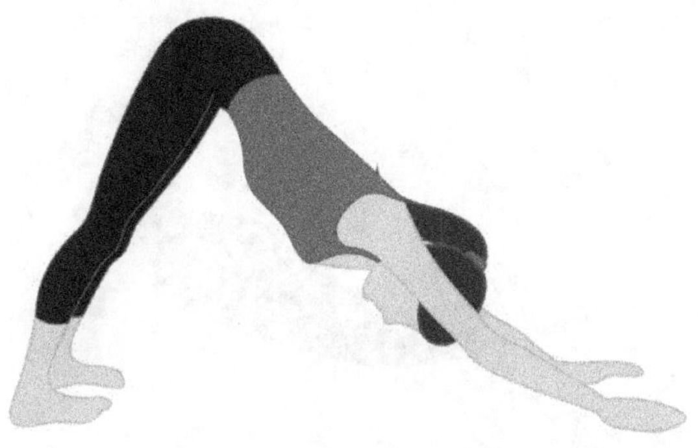

Push your right leg backwards. Keep your feet together. Bend your head and look at your navel then press your butt upwards. Feel the stretch in your legs, arms, and back. Try to keep your heels on the floor.

6. Hold your breath

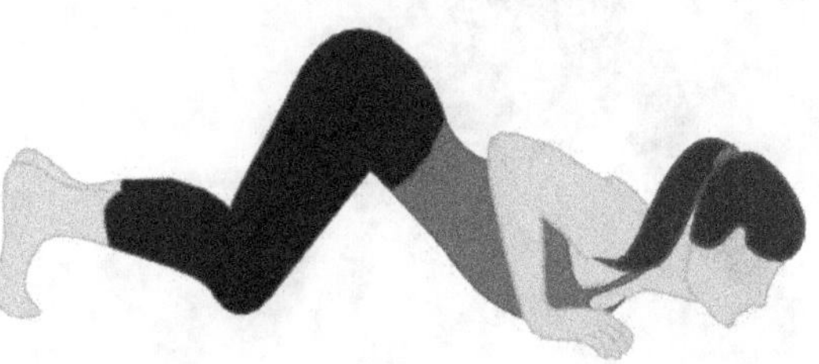

Lower your whole body through your arms against the floor in one fluid movement. Only toes, knees, chest, chin, and palms are touching the floor. Your butt must be lifted, and your elbows must point a little outward to manage the position. You will master it after a little practice.

7. Breathe in

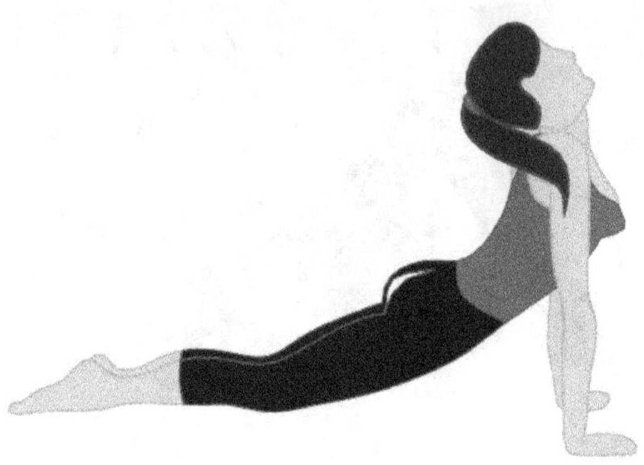

Slide forwards by pressing your upper body up with straight arms. Bend your head backwards and stretch your chin.

8. . Breathe out

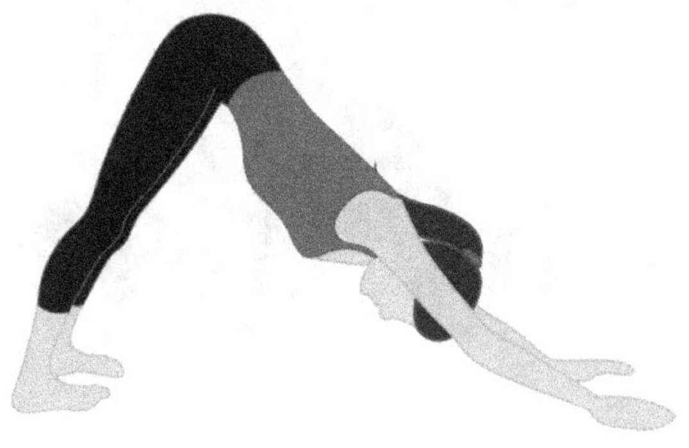

Press your butt upwards in the same position as number 5. Feet together, head towards stomach. Try to get from position 7 to 8 without adjusting your hands or feet. Your target is to slide fluidly from one position to the other with hands and feet in the same position.

9. . Breathe in

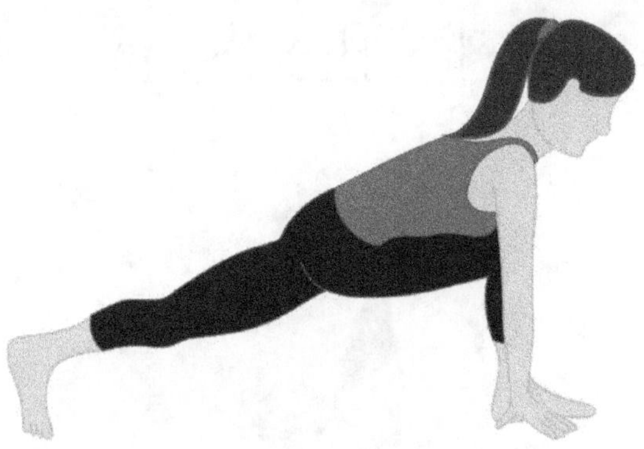

Lift your left knee forward between your arms. Same position as number 4. Remember to lift your upper body, stretch your neck and chin, and look upwards. Keep left foot at on the floor, and left knee well forward. Right knee is bent backward towards the floor.

10. . Breathe out

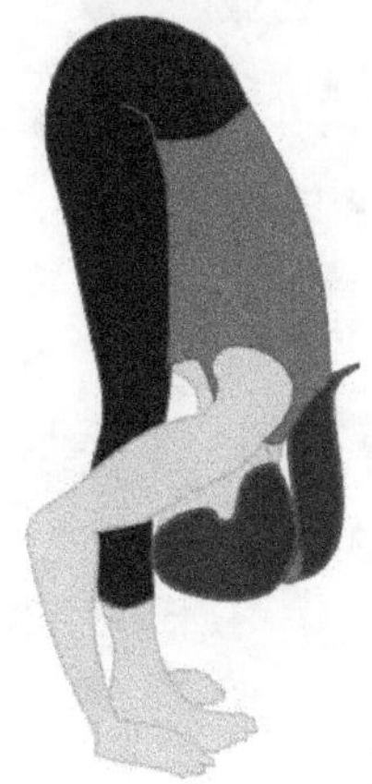

Move your right leg forward between your hands. It's the same position as number 3. Straighten up by pressing your palms to the floor (or touch with your fingertips until you are more flexible). Try to press your head toward your knees. Keep your legs straight all the time, but don´t stretch further than your body wants to. It should not be too strenuous. Take it gradually and listen to your body – it knows best.

11. . Breathe in

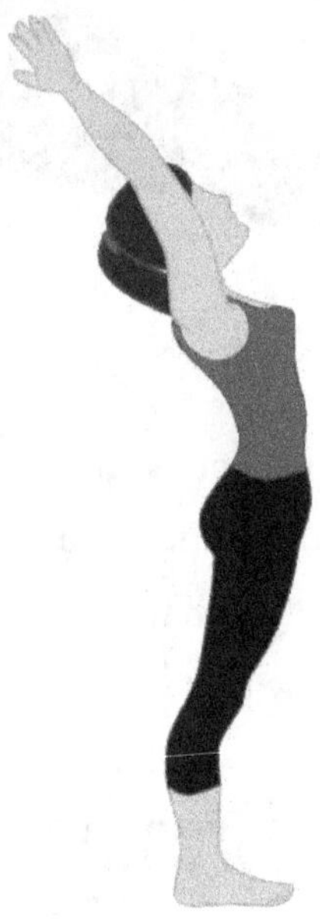

Straighten up and bend backward like in position number 2. Straight arms, locked thumbs, straight legs.

12. . Breathe out

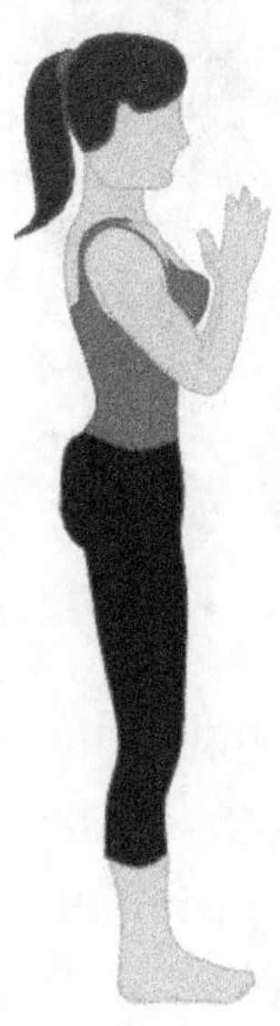

Return to your starting position with your palms together in front of your chest. Relax (or repeat the whole routine.)

Remember: This exercise benefits your whole organism, so the more repetitions you do – the better. You can also do the positions as separate exercises. Try to feel what your body needs.

When you are finished, you should lie down at on your back, and just breathe calmly while you repeat OHM, preferably chanting aloud, as it's very good for your mind and body.

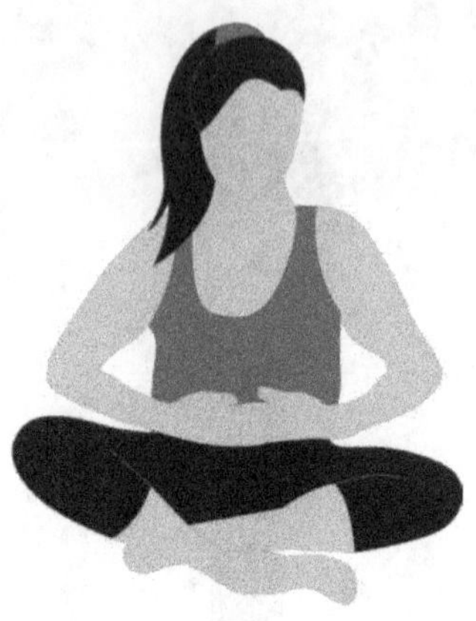

You can continue with meditation and visualization if you need stress relief and get in harmony with yourself and your surroundings. Use OHM as your mantra. It helps you to exist in the NOW.

Chapter 28

YOUR NEW LOOK

Do you get envious of the gorgeous girls you watch on the TV screen and social media? Do you get downright depressed comparing their perfect looks with the pale, ordinary face most of us see in the mirror in the early morning?

You know what? I think a lot of the screen beauties don't look so hot before they are styled either… And whatever we look like, we can do a lot to be the very best version of ourselves! The secret is to focus on your own look, not envy anybody else. Just make the most of what you have got.

One of the most important parts of your total look an image is your hair colour and style. Your hair should be your crowning glory. It's a main part of your looks and image. All of us dream of a glossy mane of healthy hair that swings like silk when we turn our head. Even if that is out of reach, at least we can get glossy, healthy hair – and find a colour and style that suits us.

You just have to find the most flattering cut and colour. You need to get a style that literally lifts and enhances your total look, with a perfect cut and in a colour that gives glow and life to your skin.

The mirror test

You can experiment a bit yourself before going to the hairdresser, just to give yourself an idea of what suits you. I think the best way is to stand in front of the mirror with no makeup and look at yourself with neutral eyes. (This is actually a trick a have learnt from a famous New York hair stylist from Brides Magazines.)

Then start rearranging your hair with your fingers, paying close attention to what makes you look better and what makes you look drab.

Will bangs make you look younger and fresher? Will it lift your face when you lift your hair upwards? Will your profile look better if your hair is cut jaw length? Do you look more stylish when you put up your hair?

Try different styles to see what suits you best and get a clear idea of what you want from your hairdresser. You can of course look in magazines and get inspired by different styles but remember that styles will differ enormously according to the quality and quantity of your hair. It will also depend on the shape of your face and the size and shape of your body.

Find your perfect style, and go for it

Really stylish women usually find their own identity and image in clothes as well as makeup and hairstyles, but they are not stuck with the same look their whole life; they adjust it according to fashion and to their age and lifestyle. Notice that most of them usually stick to classic styles, not the fancy styles that are the hairdresser favourites. The key is that the rich and famous know what suits them and they are not falling into the traps of following high street trends.

Don't chop your hair off

The worst hair blunders are - in my opinion - done by hairdressers who religiously follow new fashions in styles, cut, and colours without analyzing the client's total looks, including face shape, head shape, age, height, size, shape, hair quality, etc.

To get exactly the right hairstyle and colour, all these things must be taken into consideration. Unfortunately, a lot of hairdressers have no education in - or feeling for - style and styling. They have no clue how to make a hairstyle part of a total look. They are just focused on hair and current fashion trends in the hairdressing world.

That is why you see lots of older women who look downright horrible with short, unflattering cuts and the wrong colouring.

In my opinion, the best hairdressers are Americans because they are so good at making women look feminine and more beautiful. Of course, you can find good hairdressers and stylists everywhere; you just have to look and be very choosy. The way a hairdresser looks and behaves gives you a clue.

A first time visit to a new hairdresser should never be for a new look; it should just be for a shampoo, blow dry and to get to know the hairdresser. Ask for advice for a new style and see if it makes sense. If so, you book another appointment for your make-over. If not, thanks and by-by!

Grey or not?

When the first grey hairs appear, I think most of us feel that we are fading and, on our way, to really getting old. Even if we are just in our thirties. It's easy to cover it up, at least for some years. With all the great products for colouring at home, it's not a big deal until the grey takes over and you have to retouch all the time. This is particularly a problem for dark haired people, as their grey roots show very quickly.

The alternative is to stop the colouring and go natural, go grey, and radically change your whole appearance and in a way, your identity. Light brunettes or blondes go greyer naturally as there is less of a stark contrast in colours than for women with dark hair. Some women look great with grey hair too, and it's up to each of is to decide what's right for us.

Unfortunately, a large part of the grey-white group is ending up in the old women's club, and it's sometimes really difficult to tell them apart. In a way, they give up their identity as women, and drop into the comfort zone of low maintenance, no makeup, elastic band trousers, ugly shoes and drab colours and patterns.

You will not end up in this aging tidal wave if you choose to stay true to your female identity, your personality and keep (or rebuild) your self-confidence as an attractive mature woman with an active lifestyle and zest for life. Grey and white hair come in many shades too and can look great if you find your identity style. If in doubt, I have the following advice!

Try and see for yourself

If you have no idea what colours and style suit you, visit a wig shop! It's totally free to try on as many as you like, and you will surely find out what flatters you the most. Be realistic when you try them on and look for a length that is similar to your own hair. Also remember that the volume of the wigs is different from your own hair, but you will definitely see which shapes and shades bring out the best in you.

When you have picked out the best choices, it's a must to look at yourself in a full-length mirror from the front, the sides, and the back. Be absolutely honest and objective and find your number one hairstyle that compliments your skin tone, your size, your face, and your age.

Take selfies or ask the assistant to take some photos of you from different angles. If she wants to press you into buying, you can just tell her that you will think about it. You can also ask your partner or best friend what style they think is best for you.

Go for the best

The next step is to choose a great hairdresser. Bring in the photos and tell them exactly what you want. In many cases you must also tell them that you prefer a razor cut, not scissors with hard edges. Don't forget that a cut that looks good when the hair is wet can be disastrously short when blow dried. I always insist on deciding the exact length of the cut on dry hair. Then the hairdresser get an idea of how your hair shrinks, and it is easier to decide how much it needs to be cut to get the perfect length.

Do not let them bully you into anything else: It's your hair and your money. You are the boss and remember that modesty gets you nowhere.

Mutton dressed as lamb

I know multi-coloured hair is in fashion just now as are tattoos. When you are past 40 or more. I think you should go for more neutral, classic effects and avoid artificial colours. Remember, you are not a teenager anymore.

It looks so bad when older women try to look younger. It has exactly the opposite effect. It can be downright scary when you walk behind a person that looks like 20 from behind – and they turn around and you see a sixty plus year old face.

Try to find a colour close to your own (before it faded). Ask the hairdresser to colour it in different shades of the same nuance to make it look natural and flattering. Hints of highlights or lowlights are incredibly flattering and give lots of shine. If you want style and class, less is more.

Your wardrobe

It's better to have a few outfits that really make you look good than a wardrobe full of stuff that makes you say "I have nothing to wear". You should really try to find your style and what you look good in when it comes to colour and cut. You should have a wardrobe that is perfect for your lifestyle, not anybody else's.

If you like casual and sporty, fine. Then you find the cut and style that works for you. Classic, elegant or glamorous? As long as it's flattering for you and it makes you feel good. If you are absolutely devoid of fashion sense, you should talk to a stylist and get some basic help to find your most flattering look. You might have a good (honest) friend who can help you or perhaps children who can guide you on the right track. They are often very direct, so their advice is important. You can also surf the internet, and particularly on Pinterest you can find a lot of great wardrobe, styling and make-over tips.

To start somewhere, declutter and rearrange your wardrobe.

Get it all out and make four piles

Sort everything into four piles: Keep, maybe, give away (or sell second hand), throw away. Don´t let the maybe pile turn into a mountain. Be realistic and ask yourself:

- *What do you look good in?*

- *What do you always put back in the closet?*

- *What has been there for ages and has never been worn?*

- *What is just for happy memories of time gone past (when you were a smaller size)?*

- *What kind of underwear is unflattering and worn-out?*

- *Which shoes do you never wear because they are uncomfortable?*

- *What – what – what ....*

The most important questions are:

Am I ever going to use it again? Will it ever be flattering? Will I ever fit into it again?

Be realistic!! If you are really honest and the answer is NO, it's just taking up space and cluttering your closets. It's time to say goodbye.

Chapter 29

DETOX YOUR ENVIRONMENT

Your external environment, both at home and in the workplace (and in your car), are extensions of yourself and your aura. It's inextricably linked. If there is a wild chaos around you, it creates a wild chaos in your brain. Take control and clean up and create order in whatever you can, which will inevitably spread to your inner self.

One of the main challenges is actually the electronic addiction many have fallen victims to. The smartphones actually can make us socially very stupid people.

Electronic stress is a killer of joy and health

The blip-blip signals from our Smart Boss is making us jump to attention, wherever we are, whatever we're doing! We shift focus and look at the messages or answer the calls. This is very dangerous and part of negative stress and mental estrangement. So, my best advice for your New Lifestyle is actually to stop, think, and build some free me time into your life.

Take techno-free periods each day

Don't be available 24/7. Don't use your life for other people's lives and media junk. We spend hours every day living the lives of others, watching disasters in the far corners of the world, listening to politicians and bad sales bluffs, reading the worst news because it sells best. We become addicted because we are terrified of missing something important. We prioritize answering the phone even when we're with others. We lose focus because we have one eye and one ear on messages.

In short, technology controls us so we are completely at the mercy of it. We spend a great deal of our lives filling ourselves with useless chit-chat that doesn't benefit anyone.

Try to map how much time you spend on internet searching, checking Facebook, Twitter, Instagram, etc. and you will probably be shocked. Decide to leave your phone at home as often as you can or put it in airplane mode if you need to bring it because of children or others who need to get hold of you.

Post Corona life

Remember how strange it was during the stay-at-home Corona periods, when our social contact was just online. Remember how frustrating it was to be deprived of human closeness, touch, hugs and real contact?

Keep on remembering this extremely important lesson!

Never forget that virtual company is just a pale shadow of the real thing that we humans need to exist and be happy. Appreciate it, and make human contacts, your family and friends your number one priority.

Remember that life is too short to throw it away on useless, mindless past-times when you can have the real thing.

Go back to your thoughts in the most depressive and frightening days of the Corona pandemic. What did you think off? Who did you miss? If you should make a list of the 10 things that you considered the most important in your existence, what were they? Remember, that in all tragedies there is also the seed of solution, of inspiration to do improvements – to make it better. What are your main points for a better life?

I am sure good health ranks on top of your list.

The good thing is that your health is in your own hands, to a large degree anyway. By improving your lifestyle and your mental attitude, you can get rid of a lot of high-risk habits that can make you vulnerable and sick. You can live just a little healthier and gain a lot of advantages that will make you stronger and more resistant. You can take care of yourself in a positive way, and actually get biologically years younger instead of getting old and feeble.

What I am saying, is that your future is largely in your own hands. You have the power to decide who you will be, where and how – in the future.

Be choosy with your time

Quality is the name of the game. Take periodic media breaks. Don't sit in front of your computer endlessly scrolling and looking at stuff that is just stuff. Don't skip between TV channels and watch rubbish or endure boring movies you really don't want to see anyway.

Decide what to watch. Decide what's good for you and what makes you feel good and happy in life, and don't focus on depressive misery that you can do nothing about. It only creates frustration and bad days.

You can choose to feel good, and it doesn't matter if it's lightweight and superficial. The most important thing is how you feel.

Take a week off

Decide to put aside a week of your life when your brain and mind should not be a container for media garbage and blind brainwashing. Without media and self-selected information seeking, you will find you have lots of time.

Maybe you should put away the remote control and listen to some relaxing music. Or maybe you should be more spontaneously social and invite some good friends to a party on a weekday. Or surprise someone with a visit? Or maybe you should do something totally practical with your hands rather than just your head.

In any case, do something that is your life, not just the consideration of others. It's perhaps the most important detox cure you can follow in your life. The reward is precious time that can be used to live life for real rather than wandering around cyberspace wasting it.

When you start on your rejuvenation trip, take a good look at your surroundings! The place you live, your home, are part of your energy field.

Like plants are a reflection of the soil and the place they grow in, you are the plant that grows in your special home. If it's full of weeds, unkempt and lacks water and nutrients, the plants will look straggly and unkempt. If the garden and soil is well taken care of and there's enough sunshine and light, the same plants will look healthy, beautiful, and full of life.

Are you happy with your home?

Is your home the way you want it to be, or has it just turned out this way because you haven't had time or money to make it the home of your dreams? If it looks a bit worn and drab, you should refresh, rejuvenate, and reenergize it. Start on a plan and make your home as new as you will be.

Is it overflowing with things you have collected during a lifetime? Or stuff you haven't looked at in ages, but keep for sentimental values (or not taking the time to clear it out)?

Now is the time to rejuvenate your home too. Choose this month for a turn to a NEW LIFE that will suit you far better than the present one.

Make a plan

Visualize and write lists of what you really want! Find out what you need now and get rid of what is just taking up space that you need for better things – or just for more light and air. Don't be afraid to dream; don't be afraid that you will be lost without all the things you really never use anyway.

I can promise you that the slimming down of your possessions will make you feel lighter and happier. It's the same great feeling as getting rid of unwanted fat!

Clean up the outer mess
– it sucks your energy

Suddenly you will find more hours in your day that you can use to improve the rest of your environment. Your home is an extension of you, the most important one, and it should reflect your personality.

There is stress reduction and feel-good vibes when creating a pleasant and positive home. Very often we know what we need and want to do, but we have put it off constantly. Now, you have the time to go for it and make your home as new as you are going to be.

Feel like a new person and take control

Start with cabinets and drawers and organize so you don´t have to spend time looking for things. Focus on one room at a time and enjoy the process. Don´t be discouraged by the amount of work. Slowly, gradually, step by step will do it!

Words of wisdom from a friend's grandmother

- *Life is like a chest of drawers. If it's in total chaos, start with one drawer.*

- *Get rid of the junk and sort out the rest. Then start on the next drawer.*

- *Before you know it, all the junk you don't need is gone, and you can see what you have.*

- *You will also see what else you need, and you will feel in control. Farewell to chaos.*

Don't wait for next week

Start NOW!! It's exactly the right time to detox your home, your wardrobe, your vanity table, your bathroom drawers, your kitchen cupboards! Say farewell to clutter and get rid of everything that has lost its place and importance in your life.

Give it away, throw it away, sell it, or do whatever as long as you get it out of your new life. Start with fresh and clean spaces...

Welcome your fabulous new lifestyle

Your outside influences your inside and your inside influences your outside. The better you look, the better you feel and the more energy you get! The better your home looks, the better you feel and the prouder you are of your base. It's like smiling to the world and getting smiles back!!

If harmony reigns inside and outside you, if you take care of yourself, your health, your looks, your attitude and mind, you can say "Thank you for my wonderful life" every day when you wake up.

I sincerely hope that I have inspired you, motivated you, and given you enough information on how to renew yourself and enjoy each step of the way to a natural New You in the process.

I wish you this a wonderful life, all the best for a New You, and a lifestyle you will love and thrive on. You can follow me on Facebook, Eva Sundene – or my blog evasundene.com.

I will be so happy for comments, shares, likes, and ideas for subjects you would like me to write about.

To use a cliché: This is the first day in the rest of your life. It is time to get a fantastic new start to your new lifestyle, and I wish you all the best in transforming yourself into the most fantastic version of YOU.

Lots of love, hugs and good luck
from Eva to the new you

EXTRAS:

New You Fill in Forms

New you Body Control

Your Ideal Weight: . . . .

Your Present Dress Size: . . . .

Your Desired Dress Size: . . . .

Take your measurements on the widest part of the body area. Use the same underwear each time. Add up the weight and measurement loss each month.
The more active you are -the more muscles you get- and that will reduce your side much more than just dieting.

	Week 1	Week 2	Week 3	Week 4	Week 5	Week 6	Week 7	Week 8
Weight*	kg	kg	kg	kg	kg	kg	kg	kg
Upper arm right	cm	cm	cm	cm	cm	cm	cm	cm
Upper arm left	cm	cm	cm	cm	cm	cm	cm	cm
Bust*	cm	cm	cm	cm	cm	cm	cm	cm
Waist*	cm	cm	cm	cm	cm	cm	cm	cm
Stomach*	cm	cm	cm	cm	cm	cm	cm	cm
Hips*	cm	cm	cm	cm	cm	cm	cm	cm
Thigh right*	cm	cm	cm	cm	cm	cm	cm	cm
Thigh left	cm	cm	cm	cm	cm	cm	cm	cm
Leg right	cm	cm	cm	cm	cm	cm	cm	cm
Leg left	cm	cm	cm	cm	cm	cm	cm	cm
Ankle right	cm	cm	cm	cm	cm	cm	cm	cm
Ankle left	cm	cm	cm	cm	cm	cm	cm	cm
RESULT WEIGHT LOSS	kg	kg	kg	kg	kg	kg	kg	kg
RESULT LOSS OF	cm	cm	cm	cm	cm	cm	cm	cm

You don' t have to measure all areas every week, but do it at the beginning and once a month to track the total difference. The areas marked with a star should be measured each week.

New you Basic Food List

These are the essential foods and drinks you should stock in your kitchen.
They are really the basics for cooking.
Shop other foods once a week.
Use **NEW YOU SHOPPING LIST**.

PANTRY

- [ ] Salt (sea salt and salt with iodine)
- [ ] Black Pepper
- [ ] Garlic Powder
- [ ] Extra spices you need to buy:
- [ ] ....
- [ ] ....
- [ ] Flour
- [ ] Cornmeal
- [ ] Rice
- [ ] Pasta
- [ ] Baking soda
- [ ] Olive oil, cold pressed Virgin Oil
- [ ] Vinegar, white, red and Apple Cider
- [ ] Balsamico
- [ ] Lemon juice
- [ ] Stock (Bouillon) Cubes
- [ ] Mustard
- [ ] Sugar
- [ ] Stevia Natural Sweetener
- [ ] Jam with low sugar content
- [ ] Honey
- [ ] Eggs

DRINKS

- [ ] Coffee
- [ ] Tea - several types
- [ ] Unsweetened juice
- [ ] Fizzy water

VEGETABLES

- [ ] Onions
- [ ] Garlic
- [ ] Carrots
- [ ] Potatoes

CANNED FOODS

- [ ] Champignons
- [ ] Asparagus
- [ ] Tomatoes / Tomato sauce
- [ ] Tuna

DRINKS

- [ ] Low-fat milk
- [ ] Yogurt
- [ ] Dairy Butter

Cross off the items you need to get to have a well stocked larder.
Use it as a shopping list.

New you Shopping List

VEGETABLES & FRUIT

DIARY PRODUCTS

MEAT, FISH, FOWL

FROZEN FOODS

CANNED FOODS

BREAD & CEREALS

BASICS

SUPPLEMENTS

CLEANING PRODUCTS

OTHER HOUSEHOLD ITEMS

GO GREENER:

√ ALWAYS BRING YOU OWN SHOPPING

Other shopping tips:

√ STICK TO YOUR WEEKLY SHOPPING LIST.

√ AVOID IMPULSE SHOPPING.

√ USE CASH IF YOU ARE AN IMPULSE BUYER.

√ NEVER SHOP WHEN YOU ARE HUNGRY.

New you Natural skin & Body Care

VEGETABLE OIL, COLD PRESSED

- OLIVE OIL
- COCONUT OIL
- AVOCADO OIL
- OTHER SKIN CARE OILS

ESSENTIAL AROMATHERAPY OILS

- LAVENDER
- GERANIUM
- YLANG-YLANG
- EUCALYPTUS
- FRANKINCENSE
- OTHER ESSENTIAL OILS

Acknowledgment

For as long as I can remember, I have told myself that when I retire, I will finally have time to follow my dream and write books. It has been a long way from wanting to write this book – to making it a reality. This beautiful card from my proof-reading English friend is what finally has made it a reality.

"Just to say: Thank you so much for giving me the most amazing pleasure of being able to read and proofread your "4 weeks to a New You" book. I enjoyed every single word and am confident that it will be a best-seller and be of so much use to those who come across it. Congratulations my dearest friend. I love you very much, Katrina.xxx"

I am filled with gratitude for my wonderful life and my destiny that has brought me to this magical island of my dreams. Gratitude for my passion to write and be creative. Gratitude for fulfilling my mission of sharing my lifelong know how and expertise on lifestyle and healthy, slim living to inspire grown up women to be the best and happiest versions of themselves. I feel extremely grateful for being able to share, teach and motivate women to feel good, strong, healthy and beautiful in their own right. When I started my Shape-Up Magazine, the first lifestyle magazine for health, slimming and beauty in 1984, my slogan was: Every woman can be beautiful, she just has to know how… The concept exploded, the magazine is still alive and kicking - as am I. The pillars are still exactly the same: Nutrition. Exercise (for body and brain). Skin and body care. Inspiration and motivation.

Thank you

Emer for proof reading.

Fleur May for design and formatting.

Elin for website and blogs.

Designed by @maygraphicstudio